Recent Advances and New Perspectives in Managing Macular Degeneration

Edited by Pinakin Gunvant Davey

Published in London, United Kingdom

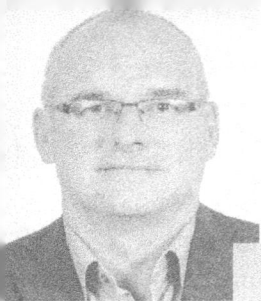
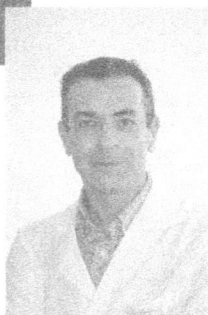
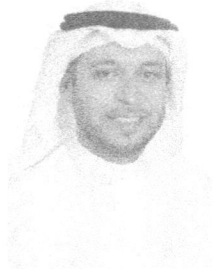
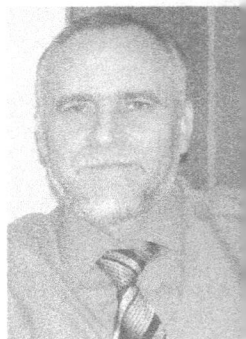
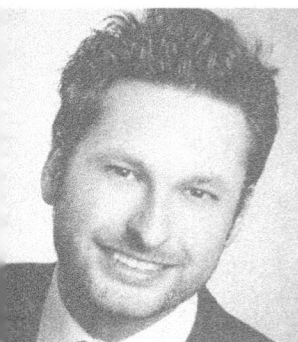
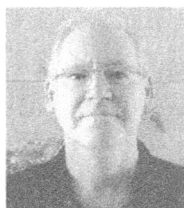
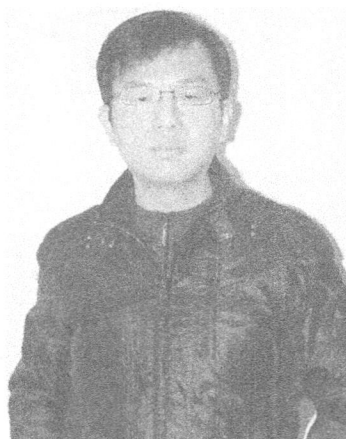

IntechOpen

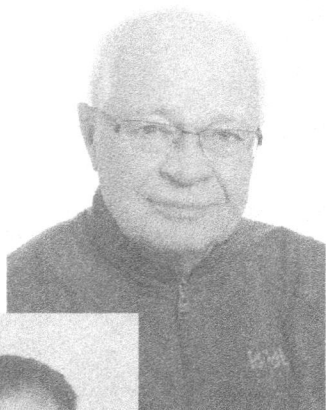
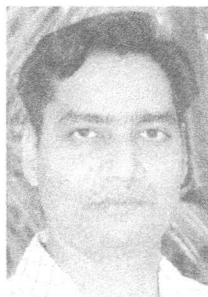
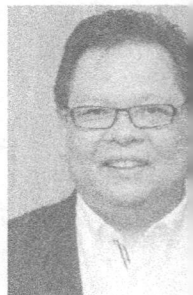
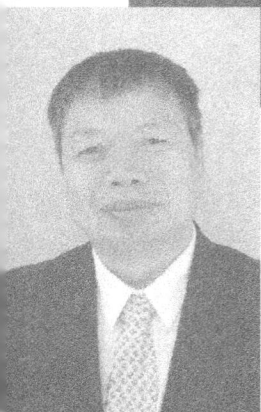
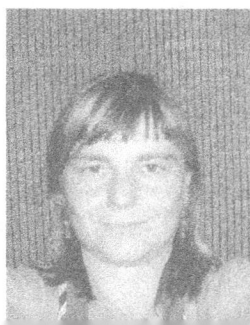
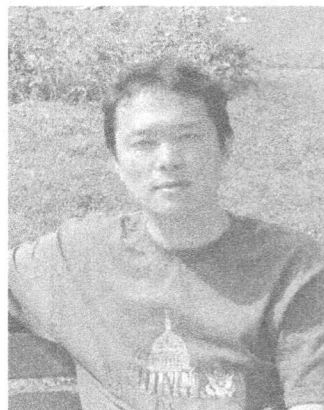

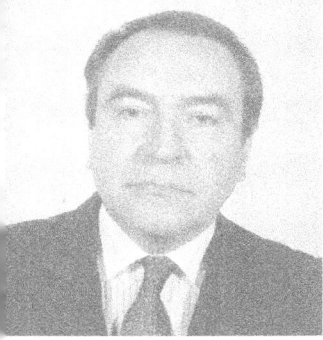

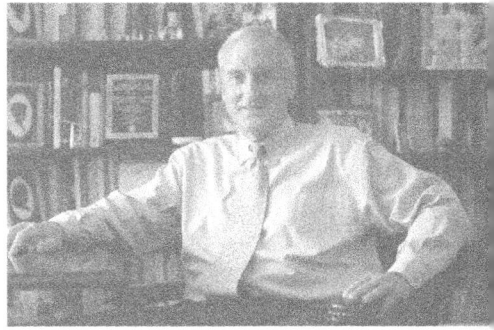

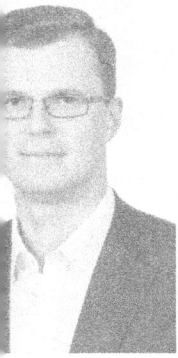

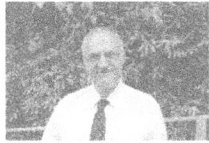

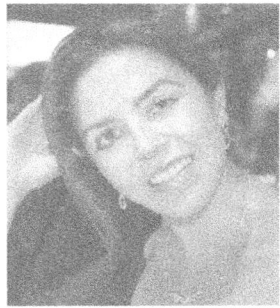

Supporting open minds since 2005

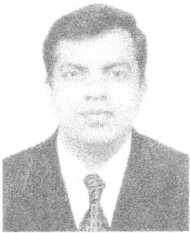

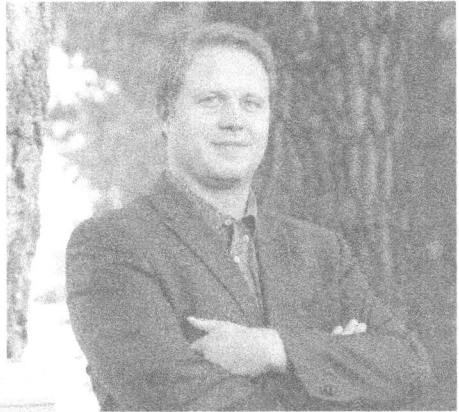

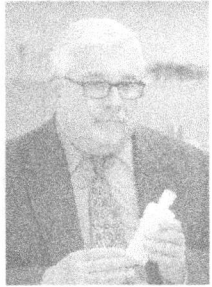

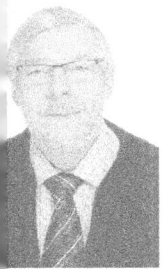

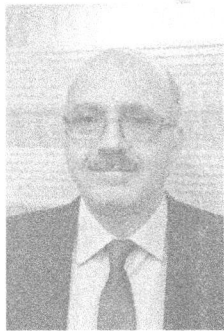

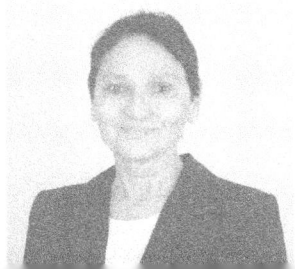

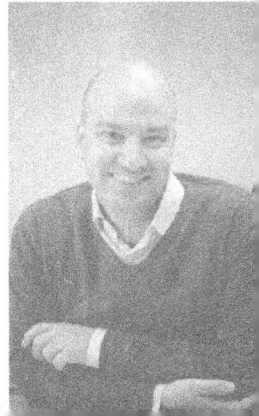

Recent Advances and New Perspectives in Managing Macular Degeneration
http://dx.doi.org/10.5772/intechopen.91530
Edited by Pinakin Gunvant Davey

Contributors
Giovanni Sato, Roberta Rizzo, Ali Hussain, Yunhee Lee, Eun Jung Ahn, Luciana de Sá Quirino-Makarczyk, Maria de Fátima Sainz Ugarte, Bernardete Pessoa, Ana Marta, Luis Leal Vega, Joaquín Herrera Medina, Adrián Martín Gutiérrez, María Begoña Coco Martin, Irene Alcoceba Herrero, Natalia Martín Cruz, Juan F. Arenillas Lara, Maja Vinković, Andrijana Kopić, Tvrtka Benašić, Pinakin Gunvant Davey, Alexander Martinez, Joseph J. Pizzimenti, Drake W. Lem

Notice
Statements and opinions expressed in the chapters are these of the individual contributors and not necessarily those of the editors or publisher. No responsibility is accepted for the accuracy of information contained in the published chapters. The publisher assumes no responsibility for any damage or injury to persons or property arising out of the use of any materials, instructions, methods or ideas contained in the book.

First published in London, United Kingdom, 2022 by IntechOpen
IntechOpen is the global imprint of INTECHOPEN LIMITED, registered in England and Wales, registration number: 11086078, 5 Princes Gate Court, London, SW7 2QJ, United Kingdom
Printed in Croatia

British Library Cataloguing-in-Publication Data
A catalogue record for this book is available from the British Library

Additional hard and PDF copies can be obtained from orders@intechopen.com

Recent Advances and New Perspectives in Managing Macular Degeneration
Edited by Pinakin Gunvant Davey
p. cm.
Print ISBN 978-1-83968-902-4
Online ISBN 978-1-83968-903-1
eBook (PDF) ISBN 978-1-83968-904-8

We are IntechOpen,
the world's leading publisher of
Open Access books
Built by scientists, for scientists

6,000+

Open access books available

146,000+

International authors and editors

185M+

Downloads

156

Countries delivered to

Our authors are among the

Top 1%

most cited scientists

12.2%

Contributors from top 500 universities

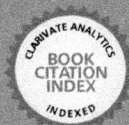

Interested in publishing with us?
Contact book.department@intechopen.com

Numbers displayed above are based on latest data collected.
For more information visit www.intechopen.com

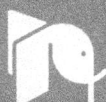

Meet the editor

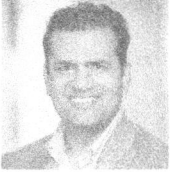

Dr. Pinakin Davey is a tenured full professor and Director of Clinical Research at Western University of Health Sciences, Pomona, California. He earned an OD from Southern College of Optometry, Memphis, Tennessee, and a Ph.D. from Anglia Ruskin University, Cambridge, England. He completed his post-doctoral research fellowship at the University of Louisville, Kentucky. His research is focused on retinal physiology and glaucoma, particularly on improving visual function in disease states. He has authored more than 75 international publications and has given more than 400 conferences and invited presentations. He serves as the vice president of the Ocular Wellness and Nutrition Society. He is also a fellow of the Association for Research in Vision and Ophthalmology (ARVO), American Academy of Optometry (AAO), and Ocular Wellness and Nutrition Society (OWNS).

Contents

Preface

Macular degeneration is one of the leading causes of blindness. The devastating effect of this blinding disease becomes more obvious as people age. Leaps and bounds of innovations and inventions have increased patient quality of life and have helped many patients regain lost vision in neovascular age-related macular degeneration (AMD). However, the therapeutic options for the more prevalent variety of macular degeneration, atrophic or "dry" AMD, are lacking.

This book is a collection of chapters that focus on the disease state of macular degeneration, issues related to the diagnosis and management of AMD, treatment considerations, and vision rehabilitation. The introductory chapter sets the tone for the book with general issues related to AMD pathogenesis. The section on diagnosis and management talks about using optical coherence tomography to aid clinical management as well as highlights the importance of discussing with patients the concept of health promotion and issues related to good diet and supplementation for atrophic AMD. The next section delves into anti-vascular endothelial growth factor therapy (anti-VEGF), which is the standard of care in AMD, and new modalities of drugs under development for the disease. One would hope that with early management and interventions we could potentially avoid the need for low vision and vision rehabilitation, but this remains an aspiration for now. Thus, the final section discusses vision rehabilitation and new strategies and advances in this area.

A multi-author edited book is never complete without contributions from experts in the field. I am grateful to all the contributing authors and the reviewers that helped shape this book. A special thanks goes to Author Service Manager Ms. Romina Rovan at IntechOpen for her tireless efforts in seeing this book to completion. Most importantly, I am grateful to my family and my dear wife Payal, and my kids Ved and Jash, who allowed me to dedicate myself to scientific pursuits. Payal, Ved, and Jash, you are truly the support that enables me to do all that I do and for that I am grateful.

Pinakin Gunvant Davey
Western University of Health Sciences,
Pomona, California, USA

Section 1

Introduction

Chapter 1

Introductory Chapter: Advances in Management of AMD

Pinakin Gunvant Davey

1. Introduction

The road from research to clinical care is a long one due to various reasons and is not entirely unjustified. In the urge for progress and "new science," one should remain vigilant in assuring that no harm is caused to the patients we serve. To this accord, the anti-VEGF therapy and the AREDS trials [1, 2] have been a game-changer in management of neovascular and atrophic macular degeneration (dry-AMD). The AREDS trials gave us evidence-based guidance on when and how to manage to prevent the progression of the disease. Whereas the neovascular AMD the vision loss is sudden, the dry-AMD the vision loss is slow and patients are unaware of the changes undergoing in their eyes. Like many other chronic diseases, dry AMD suffers from issues related to early diagnosis. The drusen that is so hallmark of dry-AMD are also seen in individuals that do not have AMD or at least not yet. How does one go about determining when the changes in retina are "normal" age-related changes or the onset of early dry AMD? The AREDS simplified grading scale [3] for AMD is a good start and the Beckman Classification System [4] improves upon the AREDS simple classification system. In the early stages of the disease dry-AMD does not show overt changes in visual function like visual acuity changes but if more challenging tasks are presented like visual function in dim illumination one indeed shows a decline. When an individual presents with a challenge in diagnosis or if the doctor would like to detect progression of the disease one could utilize extended functional testing to determine changes to visual function.

2. Functional testing and dry-AMD

Doctors have used screening color vision tests like red cap tests, Ishihara, and d-15 very successfully and they indeed have their place in our clinics. However, when investigating early visual dysfunction one may need quantifying threshold strategies. The Rabin Cone Contrast Test® is a threshold test that is helpful as an early detection strategy for various diseases. The use and benefits of color vision testing in early detection of disease and its progression is not a new concept. Numerous diseases such as diabetes cause changes to color vision prior to the onset of retinopathy [5]. The Duke University School of Medicine researchers used a variety of visual function tests and structural measurements to identify progression in early AMD and intermediate stage AMD [6]. The overarching goal was to detect progression in AMD in a short period of time and to identify useful endpoints for future clinical trials. They utilized Rabin Cone Contrast Testing® to isolate the three cone types and determine the cone contrast thresholds. This device uses precise calibration, and letter optotypes in red, blue, or green color that a patient is asked to recognize and report. This isolates and allows testing of the individual cone system's integrity whilst assuring that the other cone types are suppressed. This longitudinal study of visual function in dry-AMD showed that the Rabin cone contrast testing was able to detect changes in color vision due to progression of dry-AMD within a period 12-month [6]. These results highlight the fact that detection of progression in a short duration allows possibility for early intervention and prevention of progressive vision loss.

3. Measuring macular pigment may be key to appropriate care

One does not expect a general physician or endocrinologist to manage diabetes without blood glucose measurements or A1c values and yet eye care providers often manage dry-AMD without knowing baseline macular pigment optical density (MPOD) values. It is true that low MPOD does not mean one has AMD, but a lower MPOD is a known alterable risk factor of AMD. It is postulated that early and intermediate stages of maculopathy are predominated by oxidative stress and low-grade inflammatory activation in aging retinae [7, 8]. Thus, it is not surprising that patients with dry-AMD benefit from treatment using antioxidant therapy. The MPOD is known to vary among various ethnicities [9] and its level depends upon the dietary intake of carotenoids as they cannot be synthesized in the human body [10, 11]. The supplementation of carotenoid-vitamin therapy has indeed shown benefits in dry-AMD however these benefits are not universal [1]. There could be various reasons for the difference in benefits observed, for example, the amount of damage to the retina or bioavailability of these supplements. Given that eye is the end organ that needs to benefit from these therapies, the levels of MPOD at the fovea must increase with these therapies. The current clinical gold standard in measuring MPOD is heterochromatic flicker photometry which is a psychophysical test [10, 12]. The measurement of MPOD clinically as a baseline and during clinical follow-up allows for assessing the patient compliance to taking the nutritional supplements and assuring that the nutritional supplements are bio-available, and carotenoids are indeed reaching the end organs. The AREDS trials [1], unfortunately, did not measure MPOD. This may be due to its difficulty and inability to obtain reliable measurements as advanced stages of dry-AMD which is accompanied by less-than-optimal visual acuity.

The measurement of MPOD in poor test-takers and individuals with suboptimal visual acuity may be addressed by objective techniques of measurement of MPOD which do not depend on or require too much subjective input. There are various objective measures used in research laboratories that could provide a quick and reliable measure of MPOD. These include dual-wavelength autofluorescence techniques [13], resonance Raman imaging [14], and Macular Pigment reflectometry [12, 15]. The Macular Pigment Reflectometry not only can provide a repeatable MPOD, but also lutein and zeaxanthin optical density values [12, 15]. The MPOD values measured using the Macular Pigment Reflectometry technique closely match heterochromatic flicker photometry [12]. The measurement of an individual's lutein and zeaxanthin optical density in-vivo in a period of 30-seconds approximately offers significant clinical advantages when applied to individualized or personalized medicine. It could help answer various fundamental questions and enhance our understanding of both physiological and pathological states. When personalized medicine becomes reality, we may find that supplementing with carotenoid vitamin therapies that are needed by an individual than "one size fits all" approach may lead to better clinical outcomes.

4. Does carotenoid vitamin therapy only help intermediate stage AMD?

The AREDS trials showed that supplementation with carotenoid vitamin therapy prevented progression from intermediate to advanced stages of AMD. Further, the AREDS-2 trial [1] showed that the carotenoid supplementation with lutein and zeaxanthin indeed favored treatment, particularly in those that had low serum levels at baseline. It's a fair question to ask if the carotenoid vitamin therapy does benefit other stages of AMD? An equally important question is what other benefits can be seen in individuals with dry-AMD with carotenoid vitamin therapy? These are big questions, and it would be ideal if there were additional large-scale trials like AREDS that give us all the answers for early diagnosis, prognostic, and new treatments when they become available. This aspiration may be in part impractical for all scientific questions and when such large trials are not available doctors will need to evaluate all tiers of evidence available to derive clinical guidelines for disease states. Numerous reports have shown clinical benefits, by raising the levels of xanthophylls in the retina through dietary supplementation, thus, adjunctive carotenoid vitamin therapy may offer enhanced neuroprotection by augmenting MPOD and subsequently preventing further injury [16, 17]. Higher levels of MPOD are thought to preserve retinal tissue, specifically, the layers containing photoreceptors in the fovea, through two primary mechanisms: (1) serving as an innate optical filter against blue light; and (2) as protective antioxidants, by neutralizing free radicals and reducing consequent oxidative injury [16, 17]. In a recent systematic review of carotenoids in the management of AMD showed that there are at least 20 epidemiological studies and 35 randomized controlled trials that have evaluated this topic [17]. These studies evaluated various facets of the topic: supplementation and increase in serum carotenoids, MPOD, and changes in visual function. Whereas improvements in BCVA were seen in six out of eighteen (6/18) trials, remarkable benefits in contrast sensitivity were demonstrated in ten out of fifteen (10/15) randomized controlled trials [17]. Improvements were also seen in glare disability, photostress recovery time, and improvements in multifocal electroretinogram results [17]. Thus, it was concluded that consistent evidence from large-scale epidemiology studies, and several randomized clinical trials, substantiate the synergic neuroprotective benefits afforded by carotenoid vitamin therapy in eyes with any stage of AMD [17]. It is important to note that these visual benefits may be decreased in late-stage AMD compared to early or intermediate stage AMD [17, 18]. A dose-response relationship with stronger effect and greater serum carotenoids and MPOD levels is seen with supplementation of a greater dose of carotenoids [19]. In a recent RCT [20] we found that six-month supplementation with a greater amount of ocular carotenoids (28mg) and omega 3 supplement (675 DHA and 230 EPA), when compared to AREDS-2 formulation soft-gels (12 mg) not only provided greater serum carotenoid levels but also led to significant improvements in measured contrast sensitivity in individuals at risk of AMD. Indicating that quicker and greater visual benefits can be seen if a larger dose of ocular xanthophylls is supplemented to patients. There are numerous questions that remain to be answered for example do potent antioxidants like astaxanthin reach retinal layers? Are there any synergistic effects of these carotenoids? Scientists have answered a lot of questions and a lot more remain.

Roughly one in eight individuals aged 60 or greater is suffering from AMD; it is fair to say that it deserves our special attention. It was long believed that in the chronic disease of dry-AMD not much occurs or is needed until much later in disease state; we can confidently say, that is not true. With the advancement in clinical testing like Rabin Cone Contrast testing, we can detect this disease easily and along with devices that can measure MPOD we can better manage the disease and monitor its progression. The objective technology of Macular Pigment Reflectometry to measure MPOD, and individual carotenoid optical density shows promise in personalized medicine. Also, there is sufficient data from various RCTs to recommend carotenoid vitamin supplement at all stages of AMD, which may prevent its progression but definitely provides an improvement in vision, and who does not like an improved vision!

Author details

Pinakin Gunvant Davey
College of Optometry, Western University of Health Sciences, USA

*Address all correspondence to: contact@pinakin-gunvant.com

IntechOpen

References

[1] Age-Related Eye Disease Study 2 Research Group. Lutein + zeaxanthin and omega-3 fatty acids for age-related macular degeneration: The Age-Related Eye Disease Study 2 (AREDS2) randomized clinical trial. JAMA. 2013;**309**(19):2005-2015. DOI: 10.1001/jama.2013.4997. Erratum in: JAMA. 2013 Jul 10;310(2):208. PMID: 23644932

[2] Yin X, He T, Yang S, Cui H, Jiang W. Efficacy and safety of antivascular endothelial growth factor (Anti-VEGF) in treating neovascular age-related macular degeneration (AMD): A systematic review and meta-analysis. Journal of Immunology Research. 2022;**2022**:6004047. DOI: 10.1155/2022/6004047

[3] Age-Related Eye Disease Study Research Group, Ferris FL, Davis MD, Clemons TE, Lee LY, Chew EY, et al. A simplified severity scale for age-related macular degeneration: AREDS report no. 18. Archives of Ophthalmology. 2005;**123**:1570-1574. DOI: 10.1001/archopht.123.11.1570

[4] Ferris FL 3rd, Wilkinson CP, Bird A, Chakravarthy U, Chew E, Csaky K, et al. Beckman initiative for macular research classification committee. Clinical classification of age-related macular degeneration. Ophthalmology. 2013;**120**(4):844-851. DOI: 10.1016/j.ophtha.2012.10.036

[5] Chen XD, Gardner TW. A critical review: Psychophysical assessments of diabetic retinopathy. Survey of Ophthalmology. 2021;**66**(2):213-230. DOI: 10.1016/j.survophthal.2020.08.003

[6] Hsu ST, Thompson AC, Stinnett SS, Luhmann UFO, Vajzovic L, Horne A, et al. Longitudinal study of visual function in dry age-related macular degeneration at 12 months. Ophthalmology Retina. 2019;**3**(8):637-648. DOI: 10.1016/j.oret.2019.03.010 Epub 2019 Mar 21. Erratum in: Ophthalmol Retina. 2019 Oct;3(10):916. PMID: 31060977; PMCID: PMC6684849

[7] Beatty S, Koh H, Phil M, Henson D, Boulton M. The role of oxidative stress in the pathogenesis of age-related macular degeneration. Survey of Ophthalmology. 2000;**45**(2):115-134. DOI: 10.1016/s0039-6257(00)00140-5

[8] Xu H, Chen M, Forrester JV. Para-inflammation in the aging retina. Progress Retinal and Eye Research. 2009;**28**(5):348-368. DOI: 10.1016/j.preteyeres.2009.06.001

[9] Davey PG, Lievens C, Ammono-Monney S. Differences in macular pigment optical density across four ethnicities: A comparative study. Therapeutic Advances in Ophthalmology. 2020;**12**:2515841420924167. DOI: 10.1177/2515841420924167. Erratum in: Ther Adv Ophthalmol. 2020 Jul 8;12:2515841420943969. PMID: 32596637; PMCID: PMC7297487

[10] Bernstein PS, Delori FC, Richer S, van Kuijk FJ, Wenzel AJ. The value of measurement of macular carotenoid pigment optical densities and distributions in age-related macular degeneration and other retinal disorders. Vision Research. 2010;**50**(7):716-728. DOI: 10.1016/j.visres.2009.10.014

[11] Arunkumar R, Calvo CM, Conrady CD, Bernstein PS. What do we know about the macular pigment in AMD: the past, the present, and the future. Eye (Lond). 2018;**32**(5):992-1004. DOI: 10.1038/s41433-018-0044-0

[12] Davey PG, Rosen RB, Gierhart DL. Macular pigment reflectometry: Developing clinical protocols, comparison with heterochromatic

flicker photometry and individual carotenoid levels. Nutrients. 2021;**13**(8):2553. DOI: 10.3390/nu13082553

[13] Green-Gomez M, Bernstein PS, Curcio CA, Moran R, Roche W, Nolan JM. Standardizing the assessment of macular pigment using a dual-wavelength autofluorescence technique. Translational Vision Science & Technology. 2019;**8**(6):41. DOI: 10.1167/tvst.8.6.41

[14] Sharifzadeh M, Zhao DY, Bernstein PS, Gellermann W. Resonance Raman imaging of macular pigment distributions in the human retina. Journal of the Optical Society of America A: Optics and Image Science, and Vision. 2008;**25**(4):947-957. DOI: 10.1364/josaa.25.000947

[15] Sanabria JC, Bass J, Spors F, Gierhart DL, Davey PG. Measurement of carotenoids in perifovea using the macular pigment reflectometer. Journal of Visualized Experiments. 29 Jan 2020;(155). DOI: 10.3791/60429. PMID: 32065154

[16] Bernstein PS, Li B, Vachali PP, Gorusupudi A, Shyam R, Henriksen BS, et al. Lutein, zeaxanthin, and meso-zeaxanthin: The basic and clinical science underlying carotenoid-based nutritional interventions against ocular disease. Progress in Retinal and Eye Research. 2016;**50**:34-66. DOI: 10.1016/j.preteyeres.2015.10.003

[17] Lem DW, Davey PG, Gierhart DL, Rosen RB. A systematic review of carotenoids in the management of age-related macular degeneration. Antioxidants (Basel). 2021;**10**(8):1255. DOI: 10.3390/antiox10081255

[18] Liu R, Wang T, Zhang B, Qin L, Wu C, Li Q, et al. Lutein and zeaxanthin supplementation and association with visual function in age-related macular degeneration.

Investigative Ophthalmology & Visual Science. 2014;**56**(1):252-258. DOI: 10.1167/iovs.14-15553

[19] Ma L, Liu R, Du JH, Liu T, Wu SS, Liu XH. Lutein, zeaxanthin and meso-zeaxanthin supplementation associated with macular pigment optical density. Nutrients. 2016;**8**(7):426. DOI: 10.3390/nu8070426

[20] Davey PG, Henderson T, Lem DW, Weis R, Amonoo-Monney S, Evans DW. Visual function and macular carotenoid changes in eyes with retinal drusen-an open label randomized controlled trial to compare a micronized lipid-based carotenoid liquid supplementation and AREDS-2 formula. Nutrients. 2020;**12**(11):3271. DOI: 10.3390/nu12113271

Section 2

Diagnosis and Management

Chapter 2

OCT Biomarkers for AMD

Luciana de Sá Quirino-Makarczyk
and Maria de Fátima Sainz Ugarte

Abstract

Age-related Macular Degeneration (AMD) is an acquired retina disease that can potentially cause significant central visual impairment. Optical coherence tomography (OCT) applied to the study of retinal pathologies has revolutionized the understanding and management of AMD, especially with the technology of full-depth imaging (FDI) Spectral Domain (SD) OCT. With the increasing amount of data from several important studies using SD-OCT and OCT-angiography (OCT-A) we can now better classify and more accurately decode AMD. The purpose of this chapter is to describe the most important AMD biomarkers recently discovered using SD OCT. Understanding AMD phenotype is very important to define prognosis and individualized forms of treatment and follow up. Biomarkers on OCT have been crucial for a better understanding of AMD.

Keywords: AMD, phenotyping, OCT

1. Introduction

Age-related Macular Degeneration (AMD) is an acquired retina disease that can potentially cause significant central visual impairment. Advanced forms of the disease may present as areas of retinal pigment epithelium (RPE) loss, subretinal/sub-RPE hemorrhage or serous fluid, as well as subretinal fibrosis. Severely affected areas may have no visual function, since loss of RPE is associated with photoreceptor collapse.

When OCT (Optical Coherence Tomography) was not available yet, several studies proposed classifications using a wide variety of parameters for AMD grading systems [1–3]. In order to facilitate data comparison among those studies and develop a core grading system using color stereoscopic fundus photography, the International Age-Related Maculopathy Epidemiological Study Group compiled the results of a series of meetings among groups involved in the epidemiological analysis of Age-Related Maculopathy (ARM) [4].

Also The Macular Photocoagulation Study Group contributed significantly to AMD grading, to the understanding of natural history of subfoveal neovascularization as well as to the effectiveness of laser photocoagulation on juxtafoveal neovascularizations [5].

OCT applied to the study of retinal pathologies has revolutionized the understanding and management of AMD, especially with the technology of full-depth imaging (FDI) Spectral Domain (SD) OCT. With the increasing amount of data from several important studies using SD-OCT and OCT-angiography (OCT-A) we can now better classify and more accurately decode AMD.

The purpose of this chapter is to describe the most important AMD biomarkers recently discovered using SD OCT.

2. Cuticular Drusen

Cuticular drusen were first described by Gass in 1977 and consist of a subtype of drusen characterized by being much more numerous than small hard drusen [6]. They frequently coalesce revealing a diffuse appearance. On fluorescein angiography (FA), they are seen as a starry-sky fluorescence pattern that is most evident during the early arteriovenous phase. Some authors suggested that cuticular drusen are often initially visible in the peripheral or midperipheral retina, where the rod-to-cone ratio is the highest [7, 8]. On fundus autofluorescence (FAF), the lesions have a central hypoautofluorescent area with a rim of hyperautofluorescence. The central hypoautofluorescent area corresponds to the area of central hyperfluorescence on FA.

Based on studies with light microscopy and transmission electron microscopy, the location of cuticular drusen was determined to be at the same of hard small drusen and soft drusen: between the inner collagenous layer of the Bruch's membrane and the basal lamina of the RPE [9, 10]. Cuticular drusen are small with steep sides and contain a dense hyalinized component that is identical to hard drusen. This contrasts with soft drusen, which are larger and have sloping sides.

On B-Scan SD-OCT, cuticular drusen are located beneath the RPE and imprint the area below with a pattern of hyperreflectivity alternated with hyporeflectivity, providing an aspect similar to a barcode sign. This aspect is due to the thinning of the RPE at the apex of the drusen and thickening at the base of the drusen. On SD-OCT, the height of drusen did not correlate with the area of hyperfluorescence on FA or hypoautofluorescence on FAF (**Figure 1**).

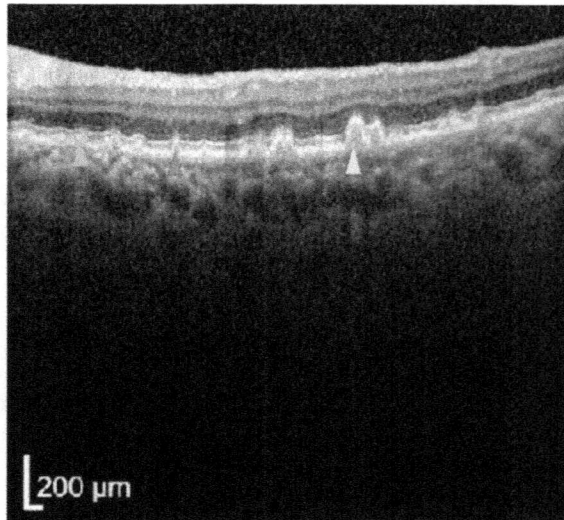

Figure 1.
Cuticular drusen. Type 1 (green arrowhead): Shallow elevations of the RPE and basal laminar band. Type 2 (red arrowhead): Triangular shape resulting in a saw-tooth appearance and hyporreflective internal contents. Type 3 (yellow arrowhead): Mound-shaped elevations of the RPE and basal laminar band with hyporreflective internal contents.

The morphological features of cuticular drusen seen on SD OCT B-scans can be categorized into 3 patterns:

1. Type 1 (33%): characterized by shallow elevations of the RPE

2. Type 2 (49%) with a triangular shape, resulting in a saw-tooth appearance, and hyporreflective internal contents

3. Type 3 pattern (18%) characterized by broad, mound-shaped elevations of the RPE with hyporreflective internal contents [11].

Near infra-red (NIR) images showed variable reflectivity patterns of cuticular drusen: hyporreflective centers with a surrounding hyperreflective margin in 53.9%, diffuse hyperreflectivity in 15.2%, heterogeneous reflectivity in 3.9%, and a combination of these patterns in 27.0%. These variations of aspects demonstrate that the accurate detection of the cuticular drusen phenotype requires the integration of data from more than one imaging method [11].

In a very extensive multimodal analysis, cuticular drusen were shown to be involved in the formation of: RPE clumping, large drusen, vitelliform lesions and subretinal neovascular membranes [11]. In the entire cohort of this study, new pigmentary RPE abnormalities were identified in 47.5% of eyes, large drusen in 45.4%, drusen resorption in 58.3% and drusen coalescence in 70.8%.

Acquired vitelliform lesions (AVL) involving the central macula were seen in 24.2% of the eyes in the study. However, visual acuity in eyes with AVLs was not significantly different from that in eyes without AVLs [11].

Geographic atrophy (GA) was identified in the macula of 25% of the eyes. The frequency of atrophy in patients older than 60 years was significantly greater than in those that were 60 years-old or younger (42.9% vs. 9.4%; $p < 0.001$). Visual acuity (VA) in eyes with atrophy was significantly worse than in those without atrophy (0.32 vs. 0.14 logMAR; $p < 0.001$) [11].

Twelve percent of the cases were complicated by choroidal neovascularization. The frequency of neovascularization in patients older than 60 years was significantly higher than in those that were 60 years-old or younger (19.6% vs. 6.2%; $p < 0.014$). The vast majority of cases (76.7%) were of type 1 neovascularization, while 9 cases were a mixture of type 1 and 2 lesions. There were no cases of type 3 macular neovascularization [11–13].

3. Reticular Drusen

Reticular pseudodrusen are multiple yellowish-white lesions arranged in a reticular network pattern. A distinction between conventional drusen and pseudodrusen was first made in 1990 by Mimoun et al. [14]. More recently the knowledge on pseudodrusen, more accurately called subretinal drusenoid deposits (SDDs), has expanded.

Reticular pseudodrusen have an increased visibility in blue light. On FAF imaging, reticular drusen are shown as numerous spots of reduced autofluorescence, with brighter lines in-between. SDDs frequently spares the fovea and usually are distributed at the superior macula, which has the highest rod-photoreceptor density [15]. Such topographic characteristic is probably related to a rod-photoreceptor association [16–18].

The fluorescein angiographic findings of subretinal drusenoid deposits are subtle, ranging from no demonstrable change to minimal hypofluorescence.

On NIR photography, reticular drusen are hyporreflective lesions, most of them with a lighter center, on a hyperreflective background. The area superior to the fovea, which has the highest rod-photoreceptor density, is the most commonly involved. The fovea, however, is typically spared [15].

The reticular pattern may not be needed for diagnosis, but most studies have required at least five reticular pseudodrusen lesions and multiple imaging modalities for confirmation of the diagnosis.

Histologic evaluation of these deposits revealed aggregation of material in the subretinal space between photoreceptors and the RPE. SDDs contain some proteins that are common to soft drusen but differ in lipid composition. There is a decrease in the number of photoreceptor nuclei above the deposits. These deposits are interconnected, forming a branching pattern [19].

SDDs contain some proteins that are common to soft drusen but differ in lipid composition.

On OCT scans, these lesions are shown as collections of granular hyperreflective deposits located between the RPE layer and the ellipsoid zone (**Figure 2**). These deposits are more commonly seen in older eyes with thinner choroids. Currently, it was shown that retinal thinning in early AMD with reticular pseudodrusen was accompanied by choroidal and retinal vascular loss, which suggests that eyes with reticular pseudodrusen may have limited compliance with changes in ocular perfusion pressure at the level of choroidal and retinal vasculature [20].

OCT has been used to classify SDD into three subtypes [21]:

1. Type 1: characterized by the presence of hyperreflective material between the RPE and the Inner/outer segment junction or ellipsoid zone (EZ). There is no elevation or breach of the EZ

2. Type 2: characterized by hyperreflective material that accumulates and forms a mound over the RPE, with distortion of overlying EZ

3. Type 3 characterized by hyperreflective material that has a conical configuration which perforates the EZ and reaches the outer retina.

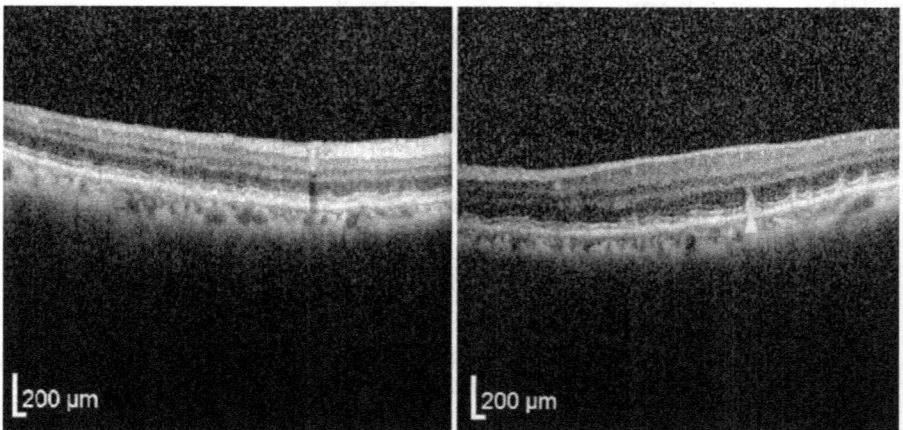

Figure 2.
Reticular drusen. The pink arrowhead indicates a stage 1 lesion where diffuse hyperreflective material between the RPE and ellipsoid layer without elevation of the ellipsoid layer. The red arrowhead indicates a stage 2 lesion with increased accumulation of hyperreflective material and distortion of the ellipsoid layer. The yellow arrowhead indicates a stage 3 lesion that has a characteristic conical shape and has punctured through the ellipsoid layer.

Many studies reported that SDDs are strong independent risk factors for late AMD. GA and type 3 neovascularization are particularly associated with SDD. Outer retinal atrophy develops in eyes with regression of SDD, a newly recognized form of late AMD [19, 22].

4. Calcified soft Drusen

This type of drusen originates from classical drusen that had their colloidal content mineralized along time. While classical drusen have a hyperreflective content due to the presence of colloid, calcified drusen have hyporreflective nodules that correspond to hydroxyapathite crystals [23].

Calcified drusen have a glistening appearance due to calcium-containing spherules and a depigmentation area around them. They present with reduced autofluorescence. On OCT, they appear as hyperreflective dots on a hyporreflective base, and they can cause shadowing of deeper structures (**Figure 3**). Refractile deposits within drusen may indicate a higher rate of GA development.

There are three calcified structures associated with advanced AMD: 1) small hyperreflective dots within drusen; [2] heterogeneous internal reflectivity within drusen (HIRD) and 3) hyperreflective lines near the Bruch's membrane. The composition of HIRD and the reason of its hyporreflectivity was not determined yet [24].

5. Subclinical Neovascular membranes

Subclinical neovascular membranes are membranes that are not exuding. Therefore, this is an important biomarker either for an exudative form or for the atrophic form of the disease.

Analyzing the NIR, B Scans and OCT-A, a neovascular complex can be observed without exudation and it is providing an elevated but shallow contour of the pigmented epithelium (**Figure 4**). The initial nomenclature of this type of membrane was quiescent neovascular membrane but more recently terminology for this finding is Shallow Irregular RPE Elevation (SIRE) [25, 26].

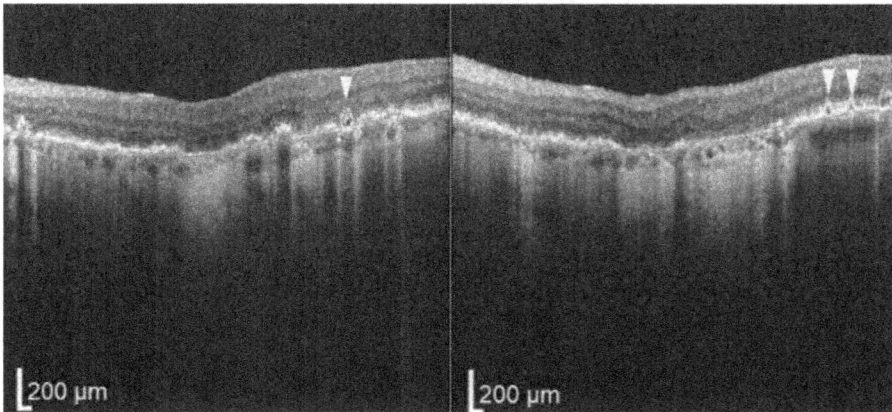

Figure 3.
Calcified small drusen (white arrowheads). In this OCT-B scan, it is possible to identify a hyperreflective sheath with a hyporreflective content. There may be hyperreflective dots inside the lesions.

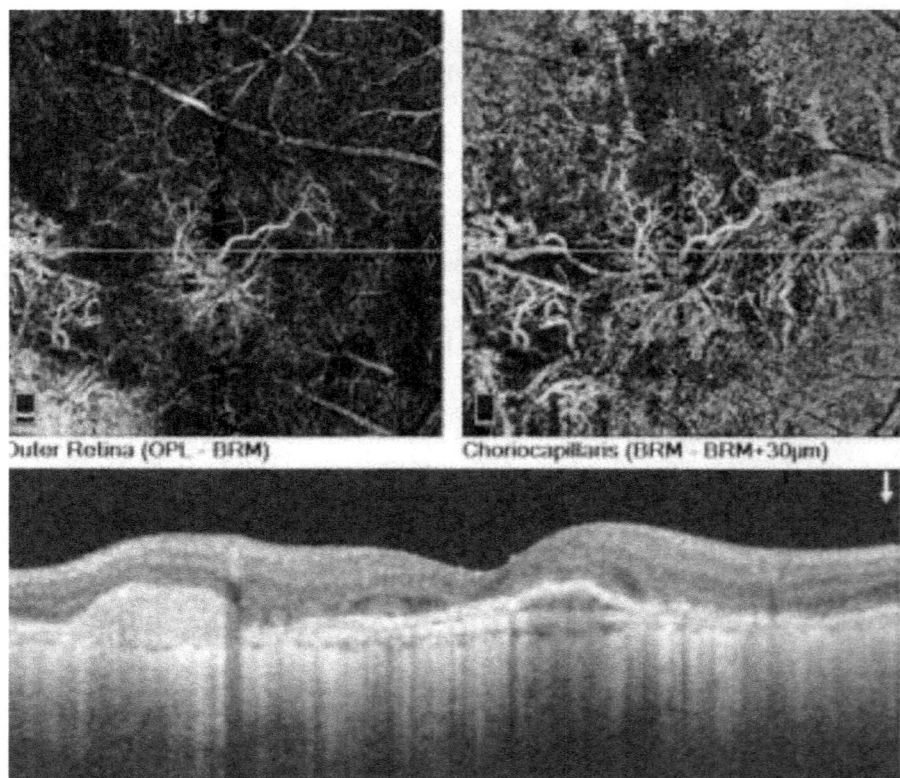

Figure 4.
SIRE. Superiorly, en face OCT-A slabs show subretinal neovascular complexes. Inferiorly, the OCT-B scan demonstrates a SIRE with the presence of heterogeneous material beneath the RPE. Additionally, it is possible to note the absence of intraretinal or subretinal fluid.

The baseline prevalence of this type of neovascularization in patients with AMD was around 13 to 14%. Exudative shift at 12 months had a prevalence of 6.8% among patients without Non-Exudative Macular Neovascularization (NE-MNV) and of 21.1% among patients with NE-MNV. Exudative shift at 24 months had a prevalence of 6.3% among patients without NE-MNV and of 34.5% among patients with NE-MNV. Therefore, it is recommendable a very close follow-up of the patients identified with SIRE [25, 26].

6. Hyperreflective foci

A concept that came to light with SD-OCTs, that we did not have previously with angiography or retinography, is intraretinal hyperreflective foci (HRF). HRF are well-circumscribed, discrete lesions with an equal or superior reflectivity compared to the RPE band on OCT (**Figure 5**). They are usually associated with hyperpigmentation on color fundus photography. There is an important specific spatial correlation of HRF with the apex of drusen [27] and/or SDD [28]. Additionally, there is an association between HRF overlying drusen and increased risk of atrophy at that location. HRF in eyes with intermediate AMD could be the result of migration of activated RPE cells into the inner retinal layers, as proposed by in vivo OCT study [29].

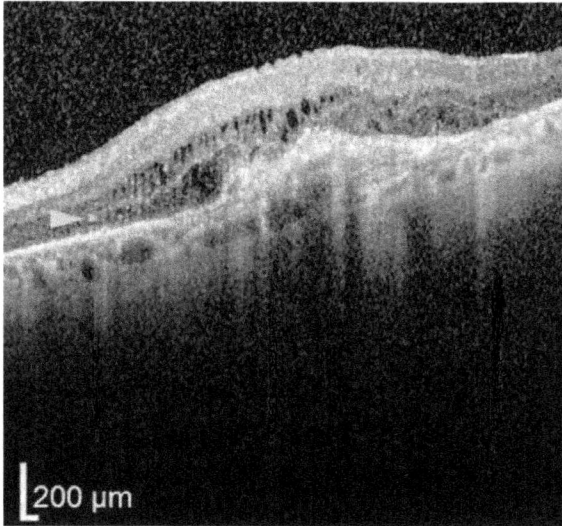

Figure 5.
Hyperreflective foci are observed in the inner (pink arrowhead) and outer retina (orange arrowhead).

Its development is triggered by a process of gliosis and phagocytosis of the Muller cells, followed by accumulation of decomposed cells in hyperreflective deposits, such as the mechanism observed in MacTel. The debris can be located at the external limiting membrane, external nuclear layer and the plexiform layer. They are biomarkers of poor prognosis, because they reveal that Muller Cells are losing their structure and will collapse [30].

Among patients classified as having intermediate AMD, the choriocapillaris flow deficit is apparently worse in eyes with HRF and is commonly located directly below HRF [31]. The amount of HRF was correlated with EZ normalized reflectivity and drusen volume (DV), that are well-defined markers of photoreceptor damage and AMD progression, respectively. Nassisi et al. [32] evaluated the correlation between HRF quantity and progression to advanced AMD after 1 year. He concluded that the area of HRF measured by en face OCT in eyes with intermediate AMD was highly correlated with development of atrophy [33, 34].

7. Acquired Vitelliform lesion

AVLs are deposits of melanosomes, melanolipofuscin, lipofuscin and outer segment debris located between the RPE and the photoreceptor layer (**Figure 6**). Their pathophysiology may be related to paraneoplastic, toxic, degenerative and vitreoretinal interface disorders of the macula.

AVL were correlated with SDD and cuticular drusen in the past and can occur in conjunction with large drusen. The same dysfunctional processes that lead to drusen formation, or parallel processes, could be related to AVL formation [35].

On fundus exam and SD-OCT, AVLs manifests as yellowish deposits between the EZ or external limiting membrane (ELM) and RPE. On FAF, they appear as areas of hyperautofluorescence that corresponded to the sites where vitelliform material was seen on SD-OCT and fundus exam. In some cases with pseudohypopyon, on FAF it is possible to identify a hypoautofluorescent top portion and a hyperautofluorescent inferior portion. On FA, there is early

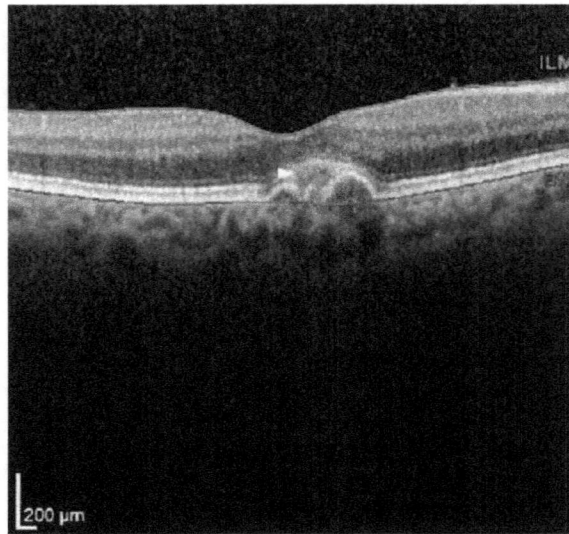

Figure 6.
Acquired Vitelliform lesion: OCT B-scan detects an accumulation of hyperreflective material between the ellipsoid layer and the RPE. This material (white arrowhead) is located above soft drusen, with discrete thinning of the overlying outer retinal layers.

hypofluorescence with a halo of hyperfluorescence. A progressive late staining of the lesion was noted during the exam. On red-free imaging studies, AVLs manifest with a slight hyperchromia of the material [36].

The lifecycle of an AVL is characterized by a phase of growth followed resorption and, over time, it can lead to complications as foveal atrophy and choroidal neovascularization (type 1 in 8% of cases). These complications are frequent and can impair central vision. There is a decrease in visual acuity from 0,3 to 0,5 logMAR (2 to 3 lines on log scale) in 7 years. Development of neovascular complexes occurs during the collapse phase of the AVL life cycle, after the AVL peak volume was reached. Type 1 choroidal neovascularization occurs in nearly 10% of cases. The risk of neovascularization and the decline in best corrected visual acuity (BCVA) are both significantly greater among eyes with AMD. Foveal atrophy was the characteristic most significantly associated with final BCVA and with change in BCVA from baseline. The development of neovascularization was not predictive of long-term visual outcomes [37].

8. Drusenoid PED

A drusenoid pigment epithelial detachment (PED) is a large elevation of the RPE that is formed from the coalescence of drusen and colloid material. It is a hallmark feature of AMD and a known precursor of GA. It may be distinguished from hemorrhagic and serous PEDs by its appearance on clinical exam and angiography (**Figure 7**). Drusenoid PEDs have an accelerated growth rate of 0,022 mm^3/month. Additionally, its rate of collapse is 10 times faster: 0,199 mm^3/month, similarly to the observed in AVL. The onset of intraretinal hyperreflective foci and AVL usually precedes its collapse.

Features such as maximal height, volume and diameter of drusenoid PEDs were inversely correlated with visual acuity and directly correlated with the rate of collapse [38].

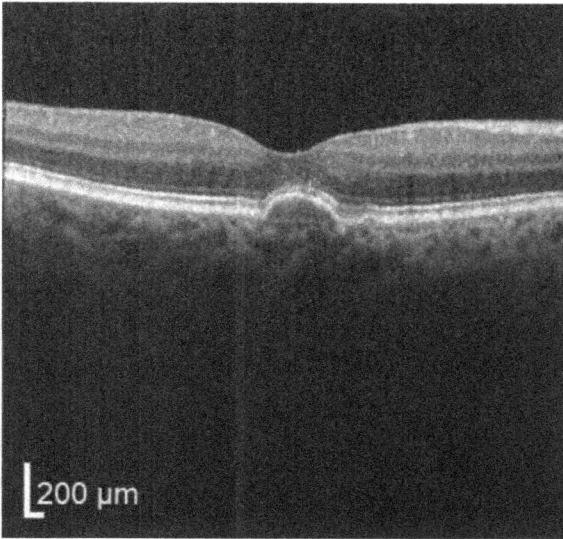

Figure 7.
Drusenoid PED. In this OCT-B scan, it is possible to note a lesion that has an internal homogenous and mild hyperreflectivity. The lesion is delimited by the Bruch's membrane at its base.

9. Macular neovascularization

In the exudative form of AMD, the local production of vascular endothelial growth factor (VEGF) promotes the growth of choroidal neovascularization. These lesions were initially classified in: classic, occult, and variations (predominantly classic and minimally classic) based on their characteristics on FA.

Gass proposed [39] that the location of the neovascular membrane could be important to predict response to treatment and after the advent of OCT, an alternative classification was suggested:

9.1 Type 1

In this type the vessels are located in the sub-RPE space (**Figure 8**). It is the most common type of neovascularization in AMD. On FA, these lesions are depicted as occult or poorly defined CNV (choroidal neovascularization). Other FA terminologies are used to describe type 1 neovascular complex: vascularized RPE, vascularized PED or stippled hyperfluorescence. On indocyanine green angiography (ICG-A), this neovascular membrane appears as an area of low-intensity hyperfluorescence, known as plaque. On SD-OCT, it is possible to determine its location on a space bounded inferiorly by the hyperreflective remnants of Bruch membrane and superiorly by the hyperreflective RPE band. A new finding of the type 1 neovascularization was described by Spaide [40] recently. It was observed that when the RPE becomes elevated due to sub-RPE exudation, the neovessels adhere to the basal surface of the RPE. On Enhanced Depth Imaging (EDI) OCT, this is described as a hyperreflective material (supposed to be the neovascularization) lining the undersurface of the elevated RPE. This pattern may explain the vulnerability of type 1 neovascularization to RPE tears. This subgroup also includes polypoidal vasculopathy, which was recently renamed as aneurysmal type 1 neovascularization.

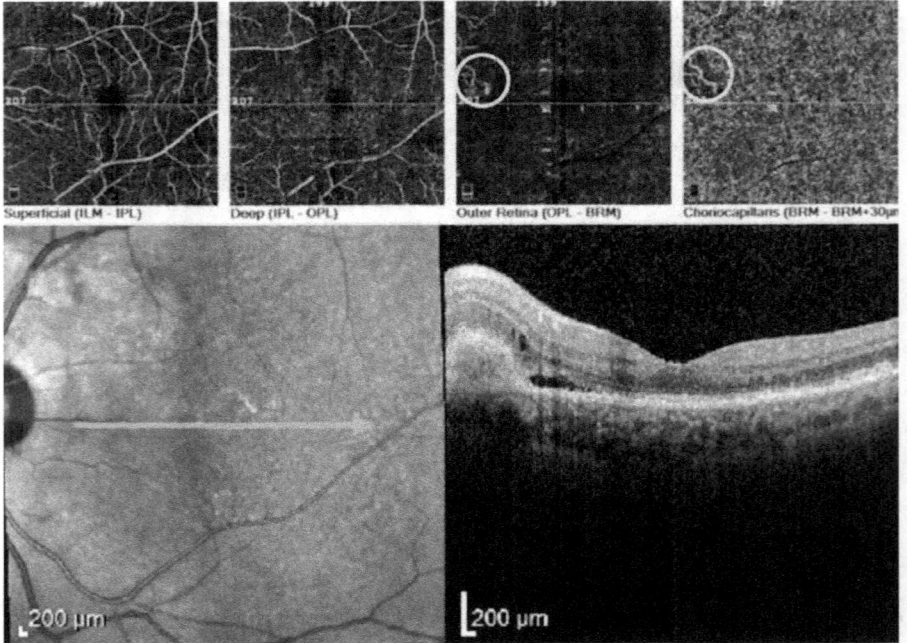

Figure 8.
Type 1 neovascularization, also known as aneurysmal type 1 subretinal neovascular membrane. Inferiorly, OCT-B scan demonstrates PED with shallow subretinal fluid and intraretinal cystic degeneration. Superiorly, OCT-A slabs detect a branch vascular network ending in an aneurysm formation (yellow circle) located between the RPE and the Bruch's membrane.

9.2 Type 2

It consists of a neovascular membrane that has perforated the RPE/Bruch membrane complex and is growing in the space between the neurosensory retina and the RPE [40]. On FA, these new vessels are commonly described as being classic or having a well-defined contour (**Figure 9**). Due to the attenuation of the choroidal fluorescence by the interjacent RPE promoting the formation of a dark background, the new vessels appear to fluoresce intensely. On the other hand, on ICG-A it may be challenging to identify the neovascular complex due to the intense hyperfluorescence of the background choroidal circulation. It is common to detect type 2 neovascularization along with type 1 vessels in exudative AMD. It is also possible that a type 2 neovascular complex regresses and turns into a type 1.

On OCT, it is possible to detect a disorganization of the overlying inner/outer segment junction in conjunction with intraretinal cystic spaces. Additionally, this exam identifies intraretinal rather than subretinal fluid.

9.3 Type 3

Type 3 neovascularization is the recent terminology for what once was known as Retinal Angiomatous Proliferation (RAP) and consists of an intraretinal neovascularization. Notable discussions happened regarding whether the origin of this neovascular complex was from the retinal circulation (as Yanuzzi suggested) or from the choroidal circulation (as suggested by Gass). Some studies support the

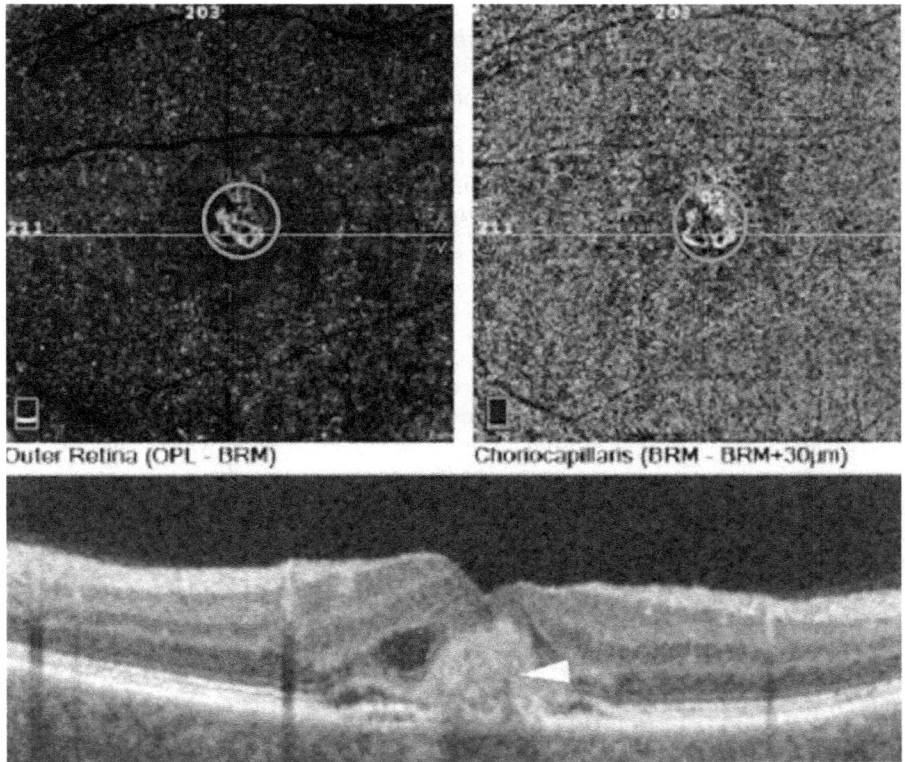

Figure 9.
Type 2 neovascularization. En face OCT-A projection images of the neovascular complex with vessels both in the outer retina and the choriocapillaris (pink circles). Inferiorly, an OCT-B scan demonstrates the neovascular complex (arrowhead) located between the RPE and the neurosensory retina.

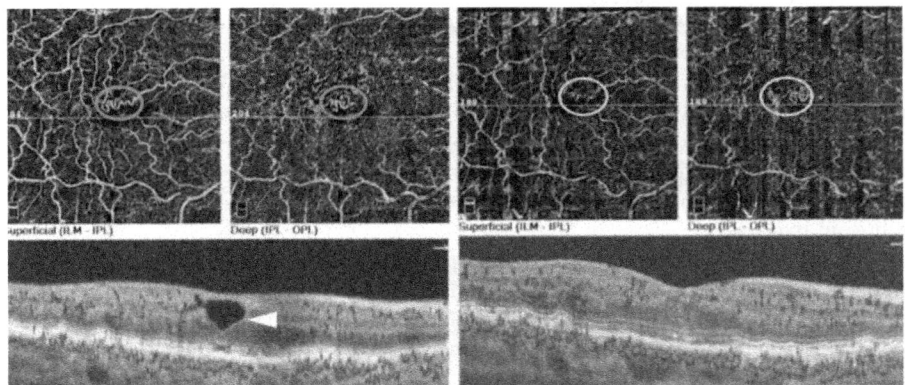

Figure 10.
Type 3 neovascularization. On the left, en face OCT-A slabs show the vascular lesion (pink circles) in the superficial and deep segments of the retina. The OCT-B scan, on the left, demonstrates the presence of intraretinal fluid, caused by the vascular lesion before treatment with anti-VEGF (arrowhead). On the right, en face OCT-A slabs still show the vascular lesion (orange circle), although the OCT-B scan, on the right, demonstrates resolution of fluid after the first injection of anti-VEGF (this type of neovascularization tends to respond well to treatment with anti-VEGF).

theory that the origin of this neovascular complex can be from either circulation and may arise from both circulations at the same time as a Retinal-Choroidal Anastomosis (RCA) (**Figure 10**).

On OCT, it is characterized by large amounts of intraretinal fluid as well as a thin choroid. In this aspect it differs from types 1 and 2 neovascularization that have an associated thickened choroid. Another differential aspect, is that type 3 neovascularization leads more often to retinal atrophy due to damage to the external retina caused by its intraretinal origin and the thinner choroid [39, 41].

10. Outer retina atrophy

Geographic Atrophy (GA) is a late-stage disease manifestation of non-neovascular AMD that generally progresses to severe central vision loss. It has traditionally been defined on color fundus photography as a sharply delineated circular or oval area of hypopigmentation or depigmentation in which choroidal vessels are visible. The size required for a lesion to be classified as GA varies with different studies, ranging from 175 μm to 430 μm in diameter.

Autofluorescence of these areas indicate them as hypoautofluorescent lesions, that may have a hyperautofluorescent rim, which is linked to acute suffering of the RPE. Atrophic areas typically demonstrate a late well-defined hyperfluorescence.

On OCT, as drusen regress, the overlying retinal layers undergo characteristic changes, while progressing to atrophy, that can be captured on OCT imaging. These changes, referred to as nascent GA in previous reports, include subsidence of the inner nuclear layer (INL) and outer plexiform layer (OPL), a hyporeflective wedge-shaped band within the Henle fiber layer (HFL), often accompanied by RPE disturbance, and increased signal hypertransmission into the choroid [42].

OCT-A shows significant impairment on the choriocapillaris flow in the zone immediately surrounding GA lesions. OCT-A seems to be able to give us information about the progression of atrophy, since the flow at the choriocapillary layer is diminished in the perifoveal region if compared to the parafoveal regions [43].

Previous studies have identified characteristic fundus features that are associated with a high risk for progression to GA [44]. Features related to a greater chance of developing GA are: large drusen volume, calcified drusen, intraretinal hyperreflective foci and SDD.

Spaide was one of the first to describe that outer retina atrophy could result from regression of SDD [45]. The outcomes of this study showed that, 43% of patients would eventually develop choroidal neovascularization after a period of two years and 43% would develop regression of SDD. Patients that had regression of SDD, had a decrease in the photoreceptor length, decrease in choroidal thickness and loss of ellipsoid band.

A score was proposed to better follow patients [28]. Among the scoring factors, there are: hyporeflective drusen, hyperreflective intraretinal foci, subretinal drusenoid deposits, and volume of large drusen. In order to generate the score, one point was assigned to each feature present in the study eye. The fellow eye was scored in a similar fashion. By adding the scores from both eyes, the total score (TS) is calculated. Category I is defined as a TS of 0, 1 or 2. Category II is defined as a TS of 3 or 4. Category III corresponds to a TS of 7 or 8. According to this score, in category I there was 0% chance to develop retinal atrophy; in category II there was a chance of 14,3%; in category III there was a chance of 47,5% and in category IV the chance was of 73%. The results allowed to conclude that patients in category I could be safely seen every 12 months, whereas patients in category II, III and IV could be seen every 6, 4 and 3 months, respectively [28, 43].

10.1 Classification of outer retina and RPE atrophy

GA usually is characterized by RPE atrophy and recently received the term RPE and outer retina atrophy (RORA). When there is a photoreceptor loss without RPE atrophy, the term proposed is outer retina atrophy (ORA). ORA also occurs in eyes after regression of reticular pseudodrusen. SD-OCT is characterized by thinning of the outer retina, including the ELM and the inner segment of the EZ band and decreased choroidal thickness. ORA increases the risk for progression to RORA or macular neovascularization [44].

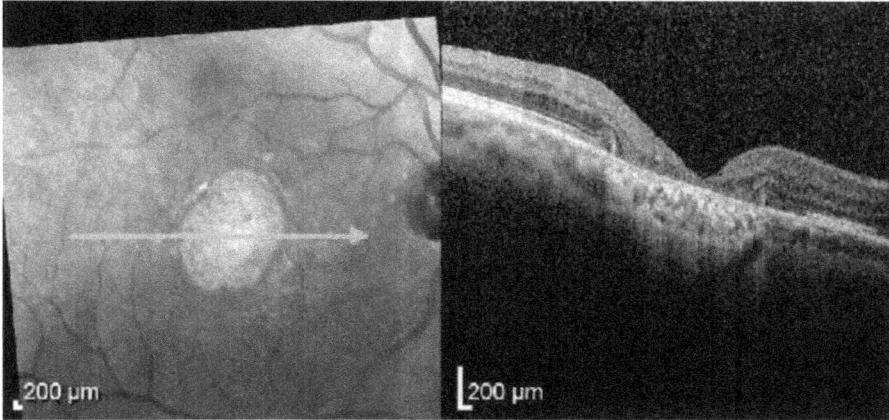

Figure 11.
cRORA. The green arrow in the red-free image, on the left, shows the location where the OCT B-scan, on the right, was taken. This scan demonstrates an area greater than 250μm in diameter with choroidal hyper-transmission due to absence of the RPE layer and overlying outer retinal thinning and loss of photoreceptors.

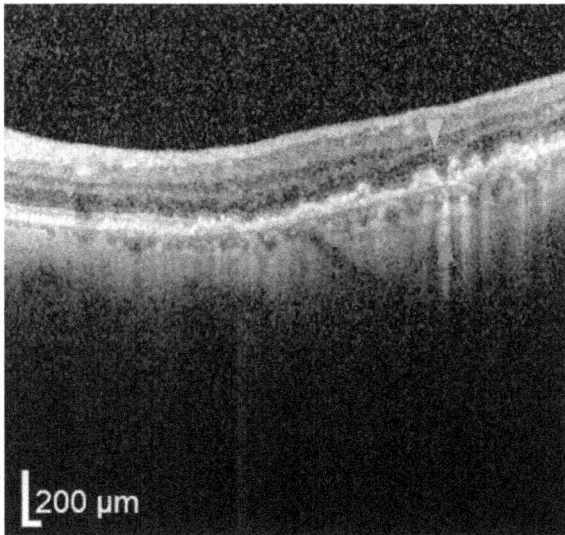

Figure 12.
iRORA. OCT-B scan demonstrates choroidal heterogeneous hypertransmission (pink arrowhead), subsidence of the INL and OPL (green arrowhead) as well as RPE attenuation and overlying photoreceptor disruption (red arrowhead).

Along several meetings, experts proposed a classification according to OCT findings and four terms were described: cRORA, complete RPE and outer retina atrophy; iRORA, incomplete RPE and outer retina atrophy; cORA, complete outer retinal atrophy and iORA, incomplete outer retinal atrophy (**Figures 11–14**) [46].

iRORA is defined on OCT by the following criteria: (1) a region of signal hypertransmission into the choroid, (2) a corresponding zone of attenuation or disruption of the RPE, with or without persistence of basal laminar deposits, and (3)

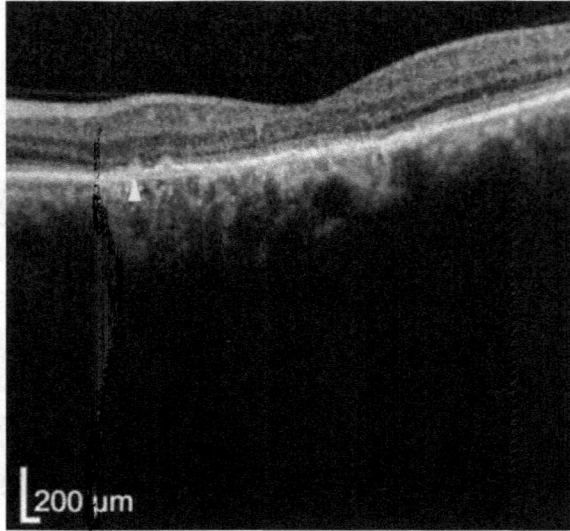

Figure 13.
cORA. OCT-B scan demonstrates thinning of the outer retina with loss of visibility of the ELM, EZ, IZ (interdigitation zone) (red arrowhead). It is possible to note regressing reticular pseudodrusen (yellow arrowhead).

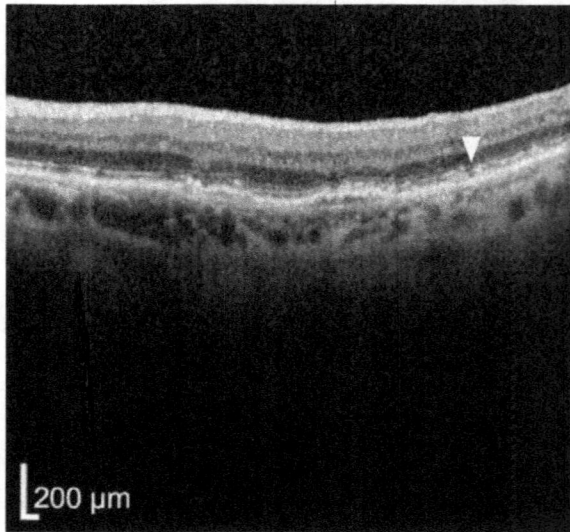

Figure 14.
iORA. OCT-B scan demonstrates thinning of the outer retina where intermittent areas of EZ and ELM can still be identified (arrowhead). It is also possible to note an uninjured RPE layer.

evidence of overlying photoreceptor degeneration (subsidence of the INL and OPL, presence of a hyporreflective wedge in the henle fiber layer (HFL), thinning of the outer nuclear layer (ONL), disruption of the external limiting membrane (ELM), or disintegration of the EZ), and when these criteria do not meet the definition of cRORA. A minimum size to determine that a lesion is iRORA was not proposed. iRORA progresses into cRORA over a variable period, from months to years. If each of the areas of RPE change and hypertransmission has a diameter of at least 250 μm on the OCT B-scan, in addition to evidence of photoreceptor loss, then they qualify as cRORA.

En face OCT allows to observe a hyperreflective contour that is the ELM descent. On FAF, this border is hyperautofluorescent. Studies have confirmed histologically that the descent ELM is an important biomarker for the development of a complete atrophy of the RPE and outer retina. Increase of ELM reflectivity also was found as possible biomarker for severe photoreceptor loss and gliosis [47–53].

Understanding AMD phenotype is very important to define prognosis and individualized forms of treatment and follow up. Biomarkers on OCT have been crucial for a better understanding of AMD.

Author details

Luciana de Sá Quirino-Makarczyk* and Maria de Fátima Sainz Ugarte
Ophthalmology Hospital of Brasília, Brasília, Brazil

*Address all correspondence to: luciana.quirino@alumni.utoronto.ca

IntechOpen

References

[1] Bressler, N. M., Bressler, S. B., West, S. K., Fine, S. L., & Taylor, H. R. (1989). The grading and prevalence of macular degeneration in Chesapeake Bay watermen. *Archives of ophthalmology (Chicago, Ill. : 1960), 107*(6), 847–852. https://doi.org/10.1001/archoph t.1989.01070010869032

[2] Gregor, Z., Bird, A. C., & Chisholm, I. H. (1977). Senile disciform macular degeneration in the second eye. The British journal of ophthalmology, *61*(2), 141–147. https://doi.org/10.1136/ bjo.61.2.141

[3] Klein, R., Klein, B. E., & Linton, K. L. (1992). Prevalence of age-related maculopathy. The Beaver Dam Eye Study. *Ophthalmology, 99*(6), 933–943. https:// doi.org/10.1016/s0161-6420(92)31871-8

[4] Bird, A. C., Bressler, N. M., Bressler, S. B., Chisholm, I. H., Coscas, G., Davis, M. D., de Jong, P. T., Klaver, C. C., Klein, B. E., & Klein, R. (1995). An international classification and grading system for age-related maculopathy and age-related macular degeneration. The International ARM Epidemiological Study Group. Survey of ophthalmology, *39*(5), 367–374. https://doi.org/10.1016/ s0039-6257(05)80092-x

[5] Laser photocoagulation of subfoveal neovascular lesions in age-related macular degeneration. Results of a randomized clinical trial. Macular Photocoagulation Study Group. (1991). *Archives of ophthalmology (Chicago, Ill. : 1960), 109*(9), 1220–1231. https://doi.org/ 10.1001/archopht.1991.01080090044025

[6] Gass JDM. Stereoscopic Atlas of Macular Diseases. Diagnosis and Treatment. 2nd ed. St. Louis: C.V. Mosby; 1977:46-50

[7] Boon, C. J., van de Ven, J. P., Hoyng, C. B., den Hollander, A. I., & Klevering, B. J. (2013). Cuticular drusen: stars in

the sky. Progress in retinal and eye research, *37*, 90–113. https://doi.org/ 10.1016/j.preteyeres.2013.08.003

[8] Boon, C. J., Klevering, B. J., Hoyng, C. B., Zonneveld-Vrieling, M. N., Nabuurs, S. B., Blokland, E., Cremers, F. P., & den Hollander, A. I. (2008). Basal laminar drusen caused by compound heterozygous variants in the CFH gene. American journal of human genetics, *82* (2), 516–523. https://doi.org/10.1016/ j.ajhg.2007.11.007

[9] Russell, S. R., Mullins, R. F., Schneider, B. L., & Hageman, G. S. (2000). Location, substructure, and composition of basal laminar drusen compared with drusen associated with aging and age-related macular degeneration. American journal of ophthalmology, *129*(2), 205–214. https://doi.org/10.1016/s0002-9394(99) 00345-1

[10] Spaide, R. F., & Curcio, C. A. (2010). Drusen characterization with multimodal imaging. Retina (Philadelphia, Pa.), *30* (9), 1441–1454. https://doi.org/10.1097/ IAE.0b013e3181ee5ce8

[11] Balaratnasingam, C., Cherepanoff, S., Dolz-Marco, R., Killingsworth, M., Chen, F. K., Mendis, R., Mrejen, S., Too, L. K., Gal-Or, O., Curcio, C. A., Freund, K. B., & Yannuzzi, L. A. (2018). Cuticular Drusen: Clinical Phenotypes and Natural History Defined Using Multimodal Imaging. Ophthalmology, *125*(1), 100–118. https://doi.org/ 10.1016/j.ophtha.2017.08.033

[12] Tan, C. S., Heussen, F., & Sadda, S. R. (2013). Peripheral autofluorescence and clinical findings in neovascular and non-neovascular age-related macular degeneration. Ophthalmology, *120*(6), 1271–1277. https://doi.org/10.1016/ j.ophtha.2012.12.002

[13] Domalpally A, Clemons TE, Danis RP, et al. (2017) Peripheral retinal

changes associated with age-related macular degeneration in the Age-Related Eye Disease Study 2: Age-Related Eye Disease Study 2 report number 12 by the Age-Related Eye Disease Study 2 Optos PEripheral RetinA (OPERA) Study Research Group. Ophthalmology, 124:479-487.

[14] Mimoun, G., Soubrane, G., & Coscas, G. (1990). Les drusen maculaires [Macular drusen]. Journal francais d'ophtalmologie, 13(10), 511–530.

[15] Klein, R., Meuer, S. M., Knudtson, M. D., Iyengar, S. K., & Klein, B. E. (2008). The epidemiology of retinal reticular drusen. American journal of ophthalmology, 145(2), 317-326.

[16] Curcio, C. A., Messinger, J. D., Sloan, K. R., McGwin, G., Medeiros, N. E., & Spaide, R. F. (2013). Subretinal drusenoid deposits in non-neovascular age-related macular degeneration: morphology, prevalence, topography, and biogenesis model. Retina (Philadelphia, Pa.), 33(2), 265–276. https://doi.org/10.1097/IAE.0b013e31827e25e0

[17] Curcio, C. A., Sloan, K. R., Kalina, R. E., & Hendrickson, A. E. (1990). Human photoreceptor topography. The Journal of comparative neurology, 292(4), 497–523. https://doi.org/10.1002/cne.902920402

[18] Zarubina, A. V., Neely, D. C., Clark, M. E., Huisingh, C. E., Samuels, B. C., Zhang, Y., McGwin, G., Jr, Owsley, C., & Curcio, C. A. (2016). Prevalence of Subretinal Drusenoid Deposits in Older Persons with and without Age-Related Macular Degeneration, by Multimodal Imaging. Ophthalmology, 123(5), 1090–1100. https://doi.org/10.1016/j.ophtha.2015.12.034

[19] Zweifel, S. A., Spaide, R. F., Curcio, C. A., Malek, G., & Imamura, Y. (2010). Reticular pseudodrusen are subretinal drusenoid deposits. Ophthalmology, 117(2), 303–12.e1. https://doi.org/10.1016/j.ophtha.2009.07.014

[20] Ahn, S. M., Lee, S. Y., Hwang, S. Y., Kim, S. W., Oh, J., & Yun, C. (2018). Retinal vascular flow and choroidal thickness in eyes with early age-related macular degeneration with reticular pseudodrusen. BMC ophthalmology, 18(1), 184. https://doi.org/10.1186/s12886-018-0866-3

[21] Zweifel, S. A., Imamura, Y., Spaide, T. C., Fujiwara, T., & Spaide, R. F. (2010). Prevalence and significance of subretinal drusenoid deposits (reticular pseudodrusen) in age-related macular degeneration. Ophthalmology, 117(9), 1775–1781. https://doi.org/10.1016/j.ophtha.2010.01.027

[22] Spaide, R. F., Ooto, S., & Curcio, C. A. (2018). Subretinal drusenoid deposits AKA pseudodrusen. Survey of ophthalmology, 63(6), 782–815. https://doi.org/10.1016/j.survophthal.2018.05.005

[23] Pilgrim, M. G., Lengyel, I., Lanzirotti, A., Newville, M., Fearn, S., Emri, E., Knowles, J. C., Messinger, J. D., Read, R. W., Guidry, C., & Curcio, C. A. (2017). Subretinal Pigment Epithelial Deposition of Drusen Components Including Hydroxyapatite in a Primary Cell Culture Model. Investigative ophthalmology & visual science, 58(2), 708–719. https://doi.org/10.1167/iovs.16-21060

[24] Tan, A. C. S., Pilgrim, M. G., Fearn, S., Bertazzo, S., Tsolaki, E., Morrell, A. P., Li, M., Messinger, J. D., Dolz-Marco, R., Lei, J., Nittala, M. G., Sadda, S. R., Lengyel, I., Freund, K. B., & Curcio, C. A. (2018). Calcified nodules in retinal drusen are associated with disease progression in age-related macular degeneration. Science Translational Medicine, 10(466), [eaat4544]. https://doi.org/10.1126/scitranslmed.aat4544

[25] de Oliveira Dias, J. R., Zhang, Q., Garcia, J., Zheng, F., Motulsky, E. H.,

Roisman, L., Miller, A., Chen, C. L., Kubach, S., de Sisternes, L., Durbin, M. K., Feuer, W., Wang, R. K., Gregori, G., & Rosenfeld, P. J. (2018). Natural History of Subclinical Neovascularization in Nonexudative Age-Related Macular Degeneration Using Swept-Source OCT Angiography. Ophthalmology, 125(2), 255–266. https://doi.org/10.1016/j.ophtha.2017.08.030

[26] Yang, J., Zhang, Q., Motulsky, E. H., Thulliez, M., Shi, Y., Lyu, C., de Sisternes, L., Durbin, M. K., Feuer, W., Wang, R. K., Gregori, G., & Rosenfeld, P. J. (2019). Two-Year Risk of Exudation in Eyes with Nonexudative Age-Related Macular Degeneration and Subclinical Neovascularization Detected with Swept Source Optical Coherence Tomography Angiography. American journal of ophthalmology, 208, 1–11. https://doi.org/10.1016/j.ajo.2019.06.017

[27] Folgar, F. A., Chow, J. H., Farsiu, S., Wong, W. T., Schuman, S. G., O'Connell, R. V., Winter, K. P., Chew, E. Y., Hwang, T. S., Srivastava, S. K., Harrington, M. W., Clemons, T. E., & Toth, C. A. (2012). Spatial correlation between hyperpigmentary changes on color fundus photography and hyperreflective foci on SDOCT in intermediate AMD. Investigative ophthalmology & visual science, 53(8), 4626–4633. https://doi.org/10.1167/iovs.12-9813

[28] Lei, J., Balasubramanian, S., Abdelfattah, N. S., Nittala, M. G., & Sadda, S. R. (2017). Proposal of a simple optical coherence tomography-based scoring system for progression of age-related macular degeneration. Graefe's archive for clinical and experimental ophthalmology = Albrecht von Graefes Archiv fur klinische und experimentelle Ophthalmologie, 255(8), 1551–1558. https://doi.org/10.1007/s00417-017-3693-y

[29] Ho, J., Witkin, A. J., Liu, J., Chen, Y., Fujimoto, J. G., Schuman, J. S., & Duker, J. S. (2011). Documentation of intraretinal retinal pigment epithelium migration via high-speed ultrahigh-resolution optical coherence tomography. Ophthalmology, 118(4), 687–693. https://doi.org/10.1016/j.ophtha.2010.08.010

[30] Echols, B. S., Clark, M. E., Swain, T. A., Chen, L., Kar, D., Zhang, Y., Sloan, K. R., McGwin, G., Jr, Singireddy, R., Mays, C., Kilpatrick, D., Crosson, J. N., Owsley, C., & Curcio, C. A. (2020). Hyperreflective Foci and Specks Are Associated with Delayed Rod-Mediated Dark Adaptation in Nonneovascular Age-Related Macular Degeneration. Ophthalmology. Retina, 4(11), 1059–1068. https://doi.org/10.1016/j.oret.2020.05.001

[31] Tiosano, L., Byon, I., Alagorie, A. R., Ji, Y. S., & Sadda, S. R. (2020). Choriocapillaris flow deficit associated with intraretinal hyperreflective foci in intermediate age-related macular degeneration. Graefe's archive for clinical and experimental ophthalmology = Albrecht von Graefes Archiv fur klinische und experimentelle Ophthalmologie, 258(11), 2353–2362. https://doi.org/10.1007/s00417-020-04837-y

[32] Nassisi, M., Fan, W., Shi, Y., Lei, J., Borrelli, E., Ip, M., & Sadda, S. R. (2018). Quantity of Intraretinal Hyperreflective Foci in Patients With Intermediate Age-Related Macular Degeneration Correlates With 1-Year Progression. Investigative ophthalmology & visual science, 59(8), 3431–3439. https://doi.org/10.1167/iovs.18-24143

[33] Ouyang, Y., Heussen, F. M., Hariri, A., Keane, P. A., & Sadda, S. R. (2013). Optical coherence tomography-based observation of the natural history of drusenoid lesion in eyes with dry age-related macular degeneration. Ophthalmology, 120(12), 2656–2665. https://doi.org/10.1016/j.ophtha.2013.05.029

[34] Leuschen, J. N., Schuman, S. G., Winter, K. P., McCall, M. N., Wong, W. T., Chew, E. Y., Hwang, T., Srivastava, S., Sarin, N., Clemons, T., Harrington, M., & Toth, C. A. (2013). Spectral-domain optical coherence tomography characteristics of intermediate age-related macular degeneration. Ophthalmology, 120(1), 140–150. https://doi.org/10.1016/j.ophtha.2012.07.004

[35] Lima, L. H., Laud, K., Freund, K. B., Yannuzzi, L. A., & Spaide, R. F. (2012). Acquired vitelliform lesion associated with large drusen. Retina (Philadelphia, Pa.), 32(4), 647–651. https://doi.org/10.1097/IAE.0b013e31823fb847

[36] Bastos, R. R., Ferreira, C. S., Brandão, E., Falcão-Reis, F., Carneiro, A. (2016). Multimodal Image Analysis in Acquired Vitelliform Lesions and Adult-Onset Foveomacular Vitelliform Dystrophy, Journal of Ophthalmology, vol. 2016, Article ID 6037537, 6 pages, 2016. https://doi.org/10.1155/2016/6037537

[37] Balaratnasingam, C., Hoang, Q. V., Inoue, M., Curcio, C. A., Dolz-Marco, R., Yannuzzi, N. A., Dhrami-Gavazi, E., Yannuzzi, L. A., & Freund, K. B. (2016). Clinical Characteristics, Choroidal Neovascularization, and Predictors of Visual Outcomes in Acquired Vitelliform Lesions. American journal of ophthalmology, 172, 28–38. https://doi.org/10.1016/j.ajo.2016.09.008

[38] Balaratnasingam, C., Yannuzzi, L. A., Curcio, C. A., Morgan, W. H., Querques, G., Capuano, V., Souied, E., Jung, J., & Freund, K. B. (2016). Associations Between Retinal Pigment Epithelium and Drusen Volume Changes During the Lifecycle of Large Drusenoid Pigment Epithelial Detachments. Investigative ophthalmology & visual science, 57(13), 5479–5489. https://doi.org/10.1167/iovs.16-19816

[39] Freund, K. B., Zweifel, S. A., & Engelbert, M. (2010). Do we need a new classification for choroidal neovascularization in age-related macular degeneration?. Retina (Philadelphia, Pa.), 30(9), 1333–1349. https://doi.org/10.1097/IAE.0b013e3181e7976b

[40] Spaide, R. F., Jaffe, G. J., Sarraf, D., Freund, K. B., Sadda, S. R., Staurenghi, G., Waheed, N. K., Chakravarthy, U., Rosenfeld, P. J., Holz, F. G., Souied, E. H., Cohen, S. Y., Querques, G., Ohno-Matsui, K., Boyer, D., Gaudric, A., Blodi, B., Baumal, C. R., Li, X., Coscas, G. J., … Fujimoto, J. (2020). Consensus Nomenclature for Reporting Neovascular Age-Related Macular Degeneration Data: Consensus on Neovascular Age-Related Macular Degeneration Nomenclature Study Group. Ophthalmology, 127(5), 616–636. https://doi.org/10.1016/j.ophtha.2019.11.004

[41] Nagiel, A., Sarraf, D., Sadda, S. R., Spaide, R. F., Jung, J. J., Bhavsar, K. V., Ameri, H., Querques, G., & Freund, K. B. (2015). Type 3 neovascularization: evolution, association with pigment epithelial detachment, and treatment response as revealed by spectral domain optical coherence tomography. Retina (Philadelphia, Pa.), 35(4), 638–647. https://doi.org/10.1097/IAE.0000000000000488

[42] Schaal, K. B., Gregori, G., & Rosenfeld, P. J. (2017). En Face Optical Coherence Tomography Imaging for the Detection of Nascent Geographic Atrophy. American journal of ophthalmology, 174, 145–154. https://doi.org/10.1016/j.ajo.2016.11.002

[43] Nassisi, M., Shi, Y., Fan, W., Borrelli, E., Uji, A., Ip, M. S., & Sadda, S. R. (2019). Choriocapillaris impairment around the atrophic lesions in patients with geographic atrophy: a swept-source optical coherence tomography angiography study. The British journal of ophthalmology, 103(7), 911–917. https://doi.org/10.1136/bjophthalmol-2018-312643

[44] Age-Related Eye Disease Study Research Group (2001). The Age-Related Eye Disease Study system for classifying age-related macular degeneration from stereoscopic color fundus photographs: the Age-Related Eye Disease Study Report Number 6. American journal of ophthalmology, *132* (5), 668–681. https://doi.org/10.1016/ s0002-9394(01)01218-1

[45] Spaide R. F. (2013). Outer retinal atrophy after regression of subretinal drusenoid deposits as a newly recognized form of late age-related macular degeneration. Retina (Philadelphia, Pa.), *33*(9), 1800–1808. https://doi.org/10.1097/IAE.0b013e 31829c3765

[46] Sadda, S. R., Guymer, R., Holz, F. G., Schmitz-Valckenberg, S., Curcio, C. A., Bird, A. C., Blodi, B. A., Bottoni, F., Chakravarthy, U., Chew, E. Y., Csaky, K., Danis, R. P., Fleckenstein, M., Freund, K. B., Grunwald, J., Hoyng, C. B., Jaffe, G. J., Liakopoulos, S., Monés, J. M., Pauleikhoff, D., ... Staurenghi, G. (2018). Consensus Definition for Atrophy Associated with Age-Related Macular Degeneration on OCT: Classification of Atrophy Report 3. Ophthalmology, *125*(4), 537–548. https://doi.org/10.1016/j.ophtha. 2017.09.028

[47] Sarks S. H. (1976). Ageing and degeneration in the macular region: a clinico-pathological study. The British journal of ophthalmology, *60*(5), 324–341. https://doi.org/10.1136/bjo.60.5.324

[48] Sarks, J. P., Sarks, S. H., & Killingsworth, M. C. (1988). Evolution of geographic atrophy of the retinal pigment epithelium. Eye (London, England), *2 (Pt 5)*, 552–577. https://doi. org/10.1038/eye.1988.106

[49] Zanzottera, E. C., Ach, T., Huisingh, C., Messinger, J. D., Spaide, R. F., & Curcio, C. A. (2016). VISUALIZING RETINAL PIGMENT EPITHELIUM PHENOTYPES IN THE TRANSITION TO GEOGRAPHIC ATROPHY IN AGE-RELATED MACULAR DEGENERATION. *Retina (Philadelphia, Pa.)*, *36* Suppl 1(Suppl 1), S12–S25. https://doi.org/10.1097/ IAE.0000000000001276

[50] Li, M., Dolz-Marco, R., Huisingh, C., Messinger, J. D., Feist, R. M., Ferrara, D., Freund, K. B., & Curcio, C. A. (2019). CLINICOPATHOLOGIC CORRELATION OF GEOGRAPHIC ATROPHY SECONDARY TO AGE-RELATED MACULAR DEGENERATION. Retina (Philadelphia, Pa.), *39*(4), 802–816. https://doi.org/10.1097/ IAE.0000000000002461

[51] Dolz-Marco, R., Balaratnasingam, C., Messinger, J. D., Li, M., Ferrara, D., Freund, K. B., & Curcio, C. A. (2018). The Border of Macular Atrophy in Age-Related Macular Degeneration: A Clinicopathologic Correlation. American journal of ophthalmology, *193*, 166–177. https://doi.org/10.1016/j.ajo. 2018.06.020

[52] Li, M., Dolz-Marco, R., Messinger, J. D., Ferrara, D., Freund, K. B., & Curcio, C. A. (2021). Neurodegeneration, gliosis, and resolution of haemorrhage in neovascular age-related macular degeneration, a clinicopathologic correlation. Eye (London, England), *35* (2), 548–558. https://doi.org/10.1038/ s41433-020-0896-y

[53] Garrity, S. T., Sarraf, D., Freund, K. B., & Sadda, S. R. (2018). Multimodal Imaging of Nonneovascular Age-Related Macular Degeneration. Investigative ophthalmology & visual science, *59*(4), AMD48–AMD64. https://doi.org/ 10.1167/iovs.18-24158

Chapter 3

Health Promotion for AMD and the Role of Nutrition

Alexander Martinez, Joseph J. Pizzimenti, Drake W. Lem and Pinakin Gunvant Davey

Abstract

There is an increase in demand for health promotion and preventative medicine playing a vital role in managing chronic illnesses. Many of these conditions stem from a poor diet, sedentary lifestyle and smoking, all of which are risk factors for age-related macular degeneration (AMD). To combat chronic diseases, the root of the conditions may be addressed through the concept of health promotion. Health promotion thoroughly assesses how a population's environmental, political, socio-economic, behavioral, and cultural practices influence its health. This concept can be applied in a primary care setting which takes on a broader approach in treating and managing patients. Primary care providers need to be aware of the connections between common chronic illnesses and AMD. All primary care providers and eyecare specialists must be patients' advocate and help improve their systemic and ocular prognosis.

Keywords: age-related macular degeneration, choroidal neovascularization, modifiable and non-modifiable risk factors, health promotion, nutrition, lutein, and zeaxanthin

1. Introduction

Age-related macular degeneration (AMD) is the leading cause of irreversible blindness in people over 50 years old [1]. It has been defined as a condition in which the structure and function of the central retina (macula) deteriorates. AMD results from a process by which the macula deteriorates over time in association with distinguishing signs and symptoms [2]. Approximately 11 million people are affected with AMD in the United States and approximately 170 million are living with AMD, worldwide [3]. In 2020, it was estimated approximately 196 million people will have AMD along with a predicted increase to 288 million by the year 2040 [4].

AMD is more commonly seen in females and individuals of Caucasian descent, especially in its late, advanced stage. Furthermore, the incidence rates vary by the stage of AMD and are related to genetics. Hispanics and Caucasians are known to have the highest incidence of early AMD. The incidence rates are 6 and 4% respectively for individuals less than fifty-five years of age which increases to 22 and 24% for individuals greater than seventy-five years of age. Overall, Asians and people of African descent show the lowest incidence of early AMD. For advanced AMD, which includes atrophic or neovascular forms, Caucasians of 75 years or older show the highest incidence at 6.5% [5].

AMD is a multifactorial disease that is influenced by age, genetics, health status, smoking habits and race [6]. With the increasing incidence of AMD secondary to a rapidly aging population, the focus is shifted on addressing modifiable risk factors like smoking cessation, altering unhealthy diets, and sedentary lifestyles [7]. AMD is the leading cause of irreversible vision loss in the developed world [8, 9]. To be proactive in addressing the rising incidence of the disease, primary care providers managing must be aware of the risk factors and associations of AMD. They are well-positioned to assist eye care professionals in preventing or slowing the progression of AMD. Primary care providers can implement a health promotion model, promoting the importance of regular eye examinations with a Doctor of Optometry or Ophthalmologists. This may enable earlier detection and treatment of AMD.

AMD is a chronic condition that currently has no known cure. Modifiable risk factors, such as an unhealthy diet, sedentary lifestyle, smoking and alcohol consumption may significantly contribute to disease onset and severity and there are successful treatment strategies [7, 10]. Health promotion is essential in reducing the risk of development and progression of AMD in high-risk groups. Health promotion also empowers patients with information, giving them control of their health. Health promotion looks into the root of the cause of the illness and assesses how environmental, political, socioeconomic, behavioral, and cultural practices influences health [11]. Primary care providers can help patients living with AMD to have a better understanding of their condition and the modifiable factors that influence their ocular and overall health. By incorporating these essential factors making up an individual's identity and influences on their health, the desired result may improve patient adherence to the management plan.

2. Methods

This is a narrative or traditional review intended to summarize the literature about health promotion for AMD and the role of nutrition. We used several databases and searches, primarily PubMed and the Cochrane Library. The principal purpose of this review is to give a comprehensive overview of the topic and to highlight significant areas of research. In addition, we seek to identify gaps in the clinical literature on health promotion for AMD and the role of nutrition and to offer information that is particularly relevant to the primary health care providers and eye care providers not specializing in the field.

3. Background

AMD affects the macular region in the retina, which is responsible for our central vision. Numerous activities such as driving, reading, cooking, operating a smart phone, and watching television depend on having a healthy macula that can be severely affected in the later stages of this condition [12, 13].

AMD can be broadly classified into two categories, as either dry AMD or wet AMD, each with their own characteristic signs and symptoms [13, 14]. AMD is graded depending on severity as early, moderate or late stage. Dry AMD's clinical features can vary depending on severity. Mild dry AMD includes few hard drusen with or without pigmentary changes in the retinal pigment epithelium (RPE) in the macular region with patients typically not complaining of any visual symptoms. The drusen (yellow deposits) are early fundoscopic signs of the disease in the macula [15, 16]. Moderate dry AMD includes one or more large drusen with or without hyperpigmentation typically associated with patients reporting visual symptoms such as persistent central blur [6]. Severe dry AMD presents with GA with significant visual symptoms and signs including reduced visual acuity, visual distortion, central visual field defects, and reduced contrast sensitivity.

AMD has a wide range of clinical presentations which correlate to the current state of the individual's visual function. Early AMD patients typically have good vision and are primarily asymptomatic or with only mild symptoms. Visual symptoms may include difficulty in dark-adapting; for example, adapting to driving at night or reading in a dimly lit room. Dark adaptation is an important biomarker of early disease [15, 17]. Moderate AMD presents with one or more large drusen the size of >125 μm in width, which is approximately the size of a branch retinal artery. This finding indicates more extensive involvement of the outer retina, the RPE, and its basement membrane [6]. Advanced AMD is associated with symptoms of reduced vision, visual distortion and central visual field defects [18].

Advanced AMD presents with clinical features of geographic atrophy (GA) and/or choroidal neovascularization (CNV). GA is a damaging clinical feature of advanced dry AMD with associated moderate to the severe reduction in vision. It presents as an area of atrophy with demarcated borders affecting the neurosensory retina which contains the photoreceptors, as well as the RPE and underlying Bruch's membrane and choriocapillaris. Presentation and size of the atrophy vary. The fovea, the central zone with in the macula, provides us with fine detail in our central vision. The foveal center is typically spared until the late stages of GA progression [19]. Approximately 20% of eyes with AMD that have progressed to legal blindness have GA as the cause. GA results from a progression of the clinical features seen in the early and moderate stages of AMD [19].

An eye with dry AMD may convert to wet AMD, where new weak blood vessels (CNV) form. CNV typically develops in the choroid and extends towards the retina causing, fluid leakage or hemorrhaging in the macular region from these new blood vessels. The natural course of untreated CNV is fibrovascular scarring, an indication of severe macular damage and profound central vision loss [18]. Patients that convert to wet AMD typically experience sudden decrease in vision along with visual distortions. Wet AMD encompasses only 10–15% of the population of patients with AMD. However, it is responsible for 80% of severe vision loss or blindness in AMD. If wet AMD is present in one eye, the fellow eye has a 48% chance of converting from dry to wet disease within 5 years. Significant risk factors for the conversion from dry AMD to wet AMD include soft confluent drusen, pigmentary irregularities and a current or past history of smoking [10].

Eyes with CNV are said to have wet AMD. GA represents large areas of cellular death. CNV represents new blood vessel growth and is associated with intraretinal, subretinal, and/or sub-RPE fluid, hemorrhage, and or scarring in the macular region. Treatment with intravitreal injection of anti-vascular endothelial growth factor (anti-VEGF) is the mainstay of treatment for active, wet AMD. This type of pharmacotherapy aims to suppress the growth of the CNV, as well as reduce the amount of associated fluid, and potentially improve vision.

3.1 Risk factors for AMD

AMD is a complex, multifactorial disease with plethora of known modifiable and non-modifiable risk factors. Modifiable risk factors include smoking, high body mass index, history of hypertension, cardiovascular disease and high alcohol consumption [20]. Smoking has consistently been proven to be a major risk factor of early AMD and late AMD in many studies [21–23]. The duration of smoking also influences the incidence of AMD, showing 14% of all AMD cases may be due to patients who smoked for 40 years [20]. Smokers have a 2 to 4-fold increase in developing AMD compared to people who do not have a history of smoking. Interestingly, former smokers who have not smoked in the last 20 years are not at a higher risk of developing AMD [20].

The literature has conflicting data from multiple studies on whether the amount of smoking or only duration increases the risk of AMD. The EUREYE study was a cross-sectional study that evaluated patients across Europe and saw a 27% correlation between smoking and the incidence of AMD [5]. Along with the increased risk of duration of smoking, the amount of cigarettes consumed and the associated increased risk of developing AMD was investigated. The Physicians' Health Study and the Nurses' Health Study determined a 2-fold increase in people who smoked 25 cigarettes per day. They also reported that males who smoked 20 or more cigarettes per day were 2.5 times more likely to develop AMD at the 12 years follow up opposed to those who did not smoke at the baseline. The Beaver Dam Study showed no association between the amount of smoking and the incidence of late AMD [24]. A meta-analysis was conducted on multiple studies that revealed a risk ratio of 2.75 for incidence of AMD when comparing current smokers versus "never smokers". When comparing former smokers versus never smokers, the risk ratio for AMD was 1.21 [5]. Smoking has also been shown to increase the incidence of the development of soft drusen and retinal pigmentary changes. Biological alterations associated with smoking increase the risk of developing AMD. For example, smoking reduces serum antioxidants, perfusion to the choroid, RPE drug detoxification pathways, and macular pigments such as lutein and zeaxanthin, further making the eye vulnerable to the development or progression of AMD [24]. Although, there is a debate if the amount of smoking during the person's smoking period is a separate risk factor, it is undeniable that a recent history of smoking does increase the risk of developing AMD.

Obesity and a sedentary lifestyle correlate with the development and progression of AMD. AMD and cardiovascular disease (CVD) have similar risk factors such as age, obesity, and smoking. Drusen in AMD and atherosclerotic plaque in CVD are relatively similar in their composition [4]. Systemic adverse effects caused by obesity include an increase in inflammatory markers, oxidative stress and blood lipid levels. These adverse effects are also factors that increase the risk for the development of AMD. This further supports the association between obesity and AMD [4]. There is also evidence for an association between obesity and low levels of the macular carotenoids lutein and zeaxanthin.

Carotenoids are fat-soluble xanthophyll pigments found throughout the retinal layers and most concentrated in the macula and are seen as a yellow spot during funduscopic evaluation. The amount and optical density of the macular pigment can be measured using clinical devices [25–31]. The macular pigment is composed of three carotenoids lutein zeaxanthin and meso-zeaxanthin an isomer of zeaxanthin. Zeaxanthin and its isomer are more concentrated than lutein within in the fovea, implying an important role for zeaxanthin in central macular integrity and the perception of fine detail [4]. Lutein's highest concentration is found in the peripheral macula. Being fat-soluble these carotenoids are also stored in adipose tissue. However, with the increase in adipose tissue in obese individuals, macular carotenoids are more readily stored in adipose tissue and are less readily available for the central retina [4, 32, 33].

A meta-analysis conducted by Zhang et al. showed a small positive association between excess body weight and risk for AMD. A low association was also found between being overweight or obese and increased risk of early AMD. This risk (for early AMD) is difficult to accurately assess because these patients are typically asymptomatic. Therefore, the association for early AMD with being overweight or obese may be underestimated in the study. Obesity was associated with an increased risk in the development of late AMD [4]. There was a linear relationship between increased body mass index and risk of AMD [4]. Therefore, the research supports a role for weight control in reducing the likelihood of developing AMD.

Obesity is a considerable public health challenge and multisystem disease. In 2009 and 2010, the prevalence of obesity was 35.5% and 35.8% in men and women in the USA, respectively [4]. The Beaver Dam Study which showed a 3.1% 15-year cumulative incidence of late AMD in adults aged 43–86 years old, so there is ultimately the potential of 110,000 cases of late AMD per year [4]. This finding is significant because obesity is a modifiable risk factor that, if addressed, can positively impact the number of AMD cases that can be avoided per year. Simply put, if the older population maintained a healthy body mass index and waist circumference, they would be giving themselves a better chance to avoid irreversible vision loss [4]. This is an example where health promotion can be effective in giving patients a strategy to avoid the development of AMD or slow its progression.

Beaver Dam Study showed the consumption of 4 or more alcoholic drinks per day was shown to increase the risk of the incidence of late AMD, specifically the wet form. It is important to note the study could not conclude heavy alcohol consumption's role in early AMD [24]. It is believed heavy alcohol consumption causes a reduction in serum antioxidants in tissues such as the retina, ultimately causing them to be susceptible to oxidative damage. Alcohol reduces the blood serum carotene, vitamin C and zinc which mirror the nutrients deficient in AMD [24].

There are risk factors for AMD that are not modifiable including age, genetics, race and sex [20]. With age the retinal layers most affected in early AMD—the RPE and underlying Bruch's membrane—begin to undergo structural and metabolic changes leading to an accumulation of metabolic waste products. Perfusion is reduced directly affecting the choroid layer that supplies nutrients to the RPE and photoreceptors (rods and cones) [5]. It is important to note that these age-related changes will not necessarily result in cellular death and functional vision loss. Environmental and genetic factors may make a person more susceptible to developing the AMD phenotype [20]. The complex integrated system of the choroid, RPE and photoreceptors contribute in maintaining the integrity of central vision. With age, this system can be altered and dysfunctional causing degenerative complications in the macula [34].

Although genetics is a known risk factor, AMD is a condition that does not follow the typical Mendelian inheritance patterns where we can predict if a relative or offspring will acquire the condition. To determine the susceptibility of a patient, the clinician has to consider the modifiable risk factors present along with the patient's age and heredity. Currently, the loci that are most associated with AMD are 1q32 (CFH) and 10q26 (PLEKHA1/ARMS2/HTRA1) [35]. Studies have shown that AMD can be present within families and show a higher incidence if a first-degree relative has been diagnosed with the disease. The Rotterdam Study showed that individuals who have a first-degree relative with AMD have a 4-fold higher risk of developing AMD [35].

3.2 Clinical diagnosis and evaluation

AMD can be diagnosed when a patient undergoes a comprehensive eye examination including dilated funduscopy by an eye care professional. The optometrist or ophthalmologist evaluates all aspects of the posterior segment of the eye, including the macula. Clinical findings associated with AMD are hard or soft drusen, retinal hypo or hyperpigmentation, macular edema, hemorrhaging and or other signs of CNV. If these findings are present, special testing can be performed to further investigate the extent of the maculopathy. Special testing includes retinal photography, autofluoresence imaging, optical coherence tomography (OCT) and fluorescein angiography. Retinal photography is used to document the appearance of the macula. Autofluoresence imaging takes advantage of the natural ability of the RPEs lipofuscin to fluoresce when stimulated with the light of a particular wavelength. It is an assessment of metabolic activity [18].

OCT is a non-invasive imaging method that uses coherent light rays to produce a cross-sectional image of the retina. OCT of the macula produces an image that shows the distinct layers of the retina and can highlight abnormalities such as macular edema, CVN, GA, and hard or soft drusen. OCT of the macula is used to further investigate any suspicious macular abnormalities in a dilated fundus exam and document the findings as a baseline reading. An OCT of the macula will then be taken at subsequent follow-ups to monitor for progression [36].

Fluorescein angiography is an invasive test involving the intravenous injection of sodium fluorescein. The dye travels to the choroidal circulation in the eye within 10–15 s, then a camera can capture images of the highlighted retinal blood circulation. Fluorescein angiography is extremely helpful in monitoring wet AMD where it can detect areas of macular edema and or active CNV [37]. It is still considered the gold standard in the detection of new CNV.

3.3 Treatment

There is currently no cure for AMD, but there are several treatments. The goal of treatment and management is to slow the progression of the disease and, in the case of wet AMD, to reduce the adverse effects of CNV. Intravitreal anti-VEGF (vascular endothelial growth factors) injections are the mainstay of contemporary therapy for active wet AMD. Lifestyle modification and nutritional supplementation have been shown to benefit patient with moderate to late dry AMD. A randomized, double-masked, placebo-controlled trial showed that people who at baseline had a lower level of macular pigment optical density (MPOD) showed benefits from taking supplements containing the dietary macular carotenoids lutein and zeaxanthin [25, 38–43]. The investigators also found an improvement in visual function associated with increased MPOD, which included visual acuity and contrast sensitivity [38, 40–43]. Increasing the macular pigment in patients appears to improve visual function and slow the progression of early AMD [38, 40–42]. However, prophylactic supplementation to prevent the onset of AMD continues to be inconclusive in the literature [40, 44].

Current management of early AMD should include health promotion with an emphasis on a healthier lifestyle involving diet, exercise and smoking cessation or avoidance. Nutrition education of patients should support the consumption of foods containing dietary macular carotenoids, which can further assist in increasing the MPOD. These foods include egg yolk, spinach, kale, collards, and brightly colored vegetables such as peppers [45]. For early AMD there is currently no treatment that can regress hard drusen or retinal pigmentary changes. A person with early AMD can continue with yearly follow-ups with their optometrist with education about lifestyle and diet/nutrition. At the initial visit, patients should be given an Amsler grid that tests the integrity of the macula. It is recommended the patient self-test each eye individually every day using their reading prescription with proper illumination to monitor their condition. The grid must be held at 33 centimeters to properly span a 20-degree field [46]. The Amsler grid test is checking for any structural changes in the macula such as new macular edema or CNV. The patient is to report whenever they notice metamorphopsia, which means the lines on the grid appear in a wavy or distorted fashion. Patients are also to report if they notice a scotoma, or missing area within the grid, and to make a timely appointment with their eye doctor.

In terms of nutritional supplementation, AREDS determined supplements may be recommended to prevent the progression of moderate AMD into late AMD [47]. These supplements contain antioxidants and micronutrients which help replenish the lack of those nutrients in the retina and consequently the properties and functions of the macula. Patients with moderate or advanced AMD need to be seen more frequently by an eye care professional than patients with early AMD. Along with the recommendation of taking the supplements listed above, reinforcing a healthier lifestyle is vital in maximizing patient outcomes.

CNV is a consequence of increased levels of VEGF in the eye. VEGF has many functions in the body including angiogenesis, bone formation, hematopoiesis, wound healing, neuroprotection and development [48]. VEGF is a potent signal protein which, when up-regulated, causes pathological angiogenesis and increased vascular permeability. For example, VEGF can give rise to new blood vessels that feed tumor growth, such as in breast cancer [48]. In AMD, the upregulation of VEGF causes the growth of new blood vessels to manifest under the RPE and/or the sensory retina. This new blood vessel growth causes devastating effects to the integrity of the macula ultimately causing a decrease in vision. Anti-VEGF therapy was initially used as cancer treatment and further investigation proved suspected beneficial ocular affects when it was noted patients' vision would also improve concurrently with cancer treatment [49].

Anti-VEGF agents are now used as a therapy for many ocular vascular diseases. The most common of these conditions are wet AMD and diabetic retinopathy. Common anti-VEGF drugs used in ophthalmic practice include bevacizumab (Avastin), ranibizumab (Lucentis) and aflibercept (Eyelea) [49]. Bevacizumab is considered an off-label therapy in retinal disease, whereas the other two drugs have an FDA indication for these purposes. Once treatment is initiated, the patient will need frequent injections to stabilize the condition along with monitoring of the macula with dilated funduscopy, OCT and fluorescein angiography [50].

4. Health promotion and prevention

Health promotion is a broad concept that looks beyond the treatment and cure of illnesses. It is a behavioral social science that looks into the biological, environmental, psychological, physical and medical sciences in order to promote health and aid in the prevention of diseases. Health promotion is effectively achieved when an individual, group, institution, or community actively engages in conversation in order to change the audience's perspective, attitude and behavior to health. Health promotion is critical due to the rippling effects it has on the improvement of overall health, reduction in premature deaths, and financial turmoil associated with medical costs for the patient and their employer. The goal of health promotion is to improve health for the individual, families, communities, cities, states and ultimately the nation. The World Health Organization (WHO) dissects health promotion into 3 elements, good governance of health, healthy cities and health literacy [51].

Good governance of health focuses on the political aspect of health promotion where local, state and federal governments play a role in their constituents' health. Ideally, the government should keep health as a main priority where they align their policies to benefit the health of its constituents. For example, these policies should focus on providing healthy school lunches for children, reducing air and water pollution, promoting exercise and general safety precautions. The WHO states when local government can focus on promoting healthy lifestyles at the municipal level it can create a healthy city with many resources. The cities can focus on community health preventions and health facilities where the local population can be screened for chronic illnesses. Health literacy is having the knowledge and understanding on how to make good choices and engage in positive habits to avoid chronic illnesses [51]. It describes how efficiently a patient can understand and monitor their disease for changes.

Health literacy is important because through disease prevention and health promotion the patient can make rational decisions when caring for their own health. A cross-sectional questionnaire study investigated whether there was an association between health literacy and chronic retinal disease [52]. The study revealed the majority of the patients with chronic retinal disease had a low level of health literacy. Sixty- five percent of patients with AMD, 73% of diabetic macular edema patients, and 63% of patients with retinal vein occlusion were shown to have low levels of health literacy.

Consequently, a low level of health literacy also influences the prognosis of the chronic retinal disease considering these conditions require self-monitoring, self-medication and self-care [52]. For example, knowing the importance of taking prescribed medicines at the appropriate dosage and time, monitoring their condition with the assigned home equipment and knowing when it is pertinent to see their provider before their scheduled appointment if new symptoms arise. Health promotion plays a major role in health literacy since these patients will be better equipped to care for their disease if properly educated. Poor health literacy is associated with poorer prognosis such as patients with uncontrolled diabetes who develop diabetic retinopathy with potential damaging effects to the retina and vision [32, 33, 52]. Another example is a patient who continues to eat unhealthy foods causing inflammation in their system, lives a sedentary lifestyle and smokes cigarettes will be more at risk for progressing to advanced AMD which causes irreversible vision loss [52].

Chronic retinal diseases demand self-management from the patient, including self-monitoring and adhering to their providers' recommendations. If this care is not maintained, vision may be negative. In order for health promotion to be effective, it must be delivered in a way the patient can grasp and understand the information. Primary care providers need to be effective communicators, avid listeners and genuinely sympathize with patient concerns. Health promotion is founded on patient-centered care with the idea health involves more than just the illness. The overall health of an individual is influenced by factors outside the health care system [11]. These outside factors include socioeconomic conditions, patterns of food consumption, demographic patterns, learning environments, and family patterns [11]. To maximize patient outcomes, the health care provider should take into consideration and include the outside factors making up the identity of the patient in their management. This approach will ultimately allow the patient to have control of their health and have a sense of responsibility to maintain it.

Health promotion has been effectively implemented with communicable infectious diseases such as sexually transmitted diseases. For example, in targeting vulnerable communities, schools held seminars where they discuss safe sexual practices and the consequences of unprotected sex such as pregnancy and sexually transmitted diseases [11]. With the increasing trend of chronic non-communicable diseases, such as hypertension, type 2 diabetes mellitus and high cholesterol, health promotion has taken a larger role in attempting to combat these conditions. The increasing incidence of these chronic conditions can be due to the increasing availability of jobs where the employees primarily work sitting at a desk in front of a computer. This type of work environment can lead to a sedentary lifestyle which is worsened when coupled with poor eating habits. In a broader view, the economy also suffers due to the widespread sedentary lifestyles that ultimately lead to chronic illnesses [11].

Other factors play a role in this health crisis such as poverty, low education and stress [11]. Consequently, these factors lead to increased risk of high blood pressure, high blood glucose, abnormal serum lipids, high waist-hip ratio, and abnormal lung function. These biological risk factors lead to chronic non-communicable diseases such as heart disease, stroke, cancer, and chronic lung disease. Therefore, health promotion is key to preventing and targeting established illnesses along with medical interventions to attain good health. Health is influenced by social, economic, political forces, cultural identities and discrepancies within communities that are more susceptible to chronic health conditions. These factors ultimately will influence the health of these vulnerable communities and their future. Thus, health promotion is vital in educating communities on the adverse effects of modifiable risk factors and the tools needed to prevent chronic conditions. An important factor of health promotion is that it allows the person to take control of their health by targeting the root of the problem that is exacerbating the illness.

5. The role of lifestyle and nutrition in AMD

AMD is a condition in which modifiable risk factors may play a significant role in its development and progression. These modifiable risk factors can be addressed through health promotion where AMD can be prevented or stabilized. Such risk factors include obesity, unhealthy diet, sedentary lifestyle, smoking, and underlying health conditions including hypertension and cardiovascular disease. A correlation between regular exercise and decreased risk in developing early or late AMD has been shown; however, the effect was stronger with lowering the progression to late AMD [53].

In general, practicing a more active lifestyle allows the person to age with less health complications in contrast to someone who is living a sedentary lifestyle. McGuiness et al. said that an active lifestyle, considered to be 3 h of moderate to intense physical activity per week, was sufficient in decreasing mortality. Regular exercise also increases antioxidant enzyme activity combating oxidative stress, avoiding the acceleration of the aging process systemically and in the eyes [53].

Regular exercise alone does not reduce the odds of developing AMD. The person must practice living a healthy lifestyle with a diet low in unhealthy foods, smoking avoidance, consuming alcohol in moderation, regular exercise and regular visits with their primary eye care and health care providers. Chronic illnesses stemming from unhealthy lifestyles have many complications and associations that include. Leading a healthy lifestyle decreases the risk of the development of chronic illnesses such as hypertension, diabetes, cardiovascular disease, and AMD [45].

Proper nutrition plays a significant role in reducing the risk of AMD. Dietary xanthophyll carotenoids play a major role in maintaining the integrity of the macula [38, 54, 55]. Seddon found that people who have a high intake of dietary carotenoids had a 43% lower risk of AMD [45]. Higher consumption of lutein and zeaxanthin correlated with a reduction in the risk of AMD. These carotenoids can be found in brightly colored vegetables as well as green leafy vegetables such as spinach, kale, turnip greens, and collard greens. Seddon's results showed that those who reported consuming a one-half cup serving of green leafy vegetables 5 times a week had an 88% reduction in the risk of AMD [45].

Another study by Seddon et al. showed evidence indicating high intake of dietary fats contributes to the progression of advanced AMD. In particular, vegetable fat was shown to increase the risk of progression of AMD. Animal fat was also shown to increase risk, but to a lesser extent [56]. The study also find that saturated, monounsaturated, polyunsaturated, and trans-unsaturated fats were remarkable for aiding the progression of AMD [56]. The results also proved dietary fat intake was independent in increasing the risk of AMD without the influence of obesity, since the participants' body mass index was controlled in the study.

Both obesity and dietary fat intake promote inflammatory markers in the body which increase the risk of cardiovascular disease and, potentially, AMD [56]. Interestingly, nuts have been shown to have a significant role in reducing the risk of cardiovascular disease, type 2 diabetes mellitus, and AMD. The Physician's Health Study showed men who consumed nuts at least twice a week had a reduction rate of 50% for the risk of sudden cardiac death and a 30% reduction rate in coronary heart disease [56]. The Nurses' Health Study revealed women who consumed nuts 5 or more times a week had a 35% reduction rate of coronary heart disease and a 27% reduction in the risk of type 2 diabetes mellitus [56]. Nuts are also said to aid in maintaining the integrity of the macula because of its beneficial properties [56]. Nuts contain resveratrol, a compound that has antioxidant, antithrombotic, and anti-inflammatory properties, which have a positive effect on the integrity of the macula [56]. Nuts also contain vitamin E, copper, magnesium, and dietary fiber which can help prevent coronary heart disease, atherosclerosis and decrease total cholesterol levels [56].

Antioxidants, vitamins and minerals have been shown to aid in reducing the risk of AMD. These micronutrients have been compounded into dietary supplements to help prevent AMD and its progression [57]. Anthocyanins, red-purple pigments, are shown to have antioxidants and anti-inflammatory properties with the potential in maintaining macular wellness [57]. Anthocyanins are found in red to purple-colored flowers, fruits and vegetables. Examples are blueberry, bilberry, strawberry, currant and grapes. Notably, bilberry has been extracted to be included in supplementation for its antioxidant properties [57]. Anthocyanins are also believed to promote the synthesis and regeneration of rhodopsin, along with promoting an increase in blood flow in the retina.

The xanthophylls lutein and zeaxanthin are carotenoids that are only obtained through the diet since the body is unable to synthesize them. Lutein and zeaxanthin are found in green leafy vegetables, such as spinach and kale, along with fruits avocado and maize [45, 57]. Lutein and zeaxanthin are most concentrated within the macula. The retinal isomerases convert lutein into meso-zeaxanthin in the retina which is also found in macula [58]. The MPOD value directly correlates with the integrity of the macula. The macular carotenoids begin to degenerate when an individual lives an unhealthy lifestyle, consequently increasing inflammatory markers. Individuals at risk for AMD or with signs of the disease may benefit from foods with lutein and zeaxanthin or supplementation with these to increase their serum and macular carotenoid levels. An increase in lutein and zeaxanthin serum levels secondary to supplementation has been shown to increase MPOD and improve visual function measures such as contrast sensitivity, glare tolerance and photo stress recovery [40–42, 57, 59, 60].

Vitamins A, C and E are micronutrients that have been shown to reduce the risk of AMD [57]. Fruits and vegetables rich in vitamin A have shown a strong association with a decreased risk of AMD due to vitamins A's close relationship to carotenoids. Vitamin C is a potent antioxidant that protects the body from free radicals causing oxidative stress. Deprived levels of vitamin C can cause an accumulation of lipofuscin and loss of photoreceptors [57]. Vitamin E is also a potent antioxidant and serves as an important micronutrient in regulating retinal health. Zinc is a mineral that serves as a co-factor for metabolically active enzymes which has many vital roles in maintaining immunity, reproduction and neuronal development. Zinc is also found in the retina where it serves a vital role in maintaining macular health [57].

Bioavailability is an important factor to consider, since the absorption of micronutrients is affected by multiple factors such as stress, alcohol consumption, caffeine, drug intake, and exercise [57]. Fats and oils have been shown to assist in the absorption of these micronutrients. With that in mind, obtaining these micronutrients from animal sources rather than plant-based sources can increase their absorption. For example, egg yolk is an excellent source of zeaxanthin and has shown to be more bioavailable than comparable amounts from oral supplements or from plant sources [57].

5.1 AREDS-1, AREDS-2 and the Rotterdam study

Before the age-related eye disease study (AREDS), supplements containing zinc and antioxidants for AMD prevention and treatment were available for consumer consumption despite little evidence of its effects on risk reduction [61]. Therefore, the National Eye Institute (NEI) developed a randomized clinical trial where high doses of zinc and antioxidant vitamins (vitamins C, E and beta carotene) were investigated. AREDS was an 11-center double-masked clinical trial. The subjects were divided into 4 groups and had to have vision of 20/32 or better in one eye [61]. The first group was randomized to take a formula consisting of 500 mg of vitamin C, 400 IU of vitamin E, and 15 mg of beta carotene. The second was assigned to take mineral supplements of 80 mg of zinc, as zinc oxide and 2 mg of copper as cupric oxide. The third group was placed on a combination of both antioxidants and zinc while the fourth group took a placebo [61].

The results of AREDS showed that the group taking antioxidants plus zinc had the highest odds reduction, odds ratio (OR) of 0.66, along with a 25% risk reduction in AMD [47]. The AREDS study concluded that people aged 55 years or older with moderate AMD (defined as the presence of one or more of the following: extensive intermediate size drusen, at least 1 large druse, or non-central geographic atrophy in 1 or both eyes) or advanced AMD or vision loss due to AMD in 1 eye (but not the other), and without contraindications such as smoking, should consider taking a supplement of antioxidants plus zinc. In contrast to eyes with early AMD, which did not benefit from supplementation, people with intermediate to advanced AMD showed a greater effect in reducing the risk of progressing while taking antioxidants and zinc supplements [47].

AREDS 2 was a multicenter, randomized, double-masked, placebo-controlled phase 3 study that investigated whether the carotenoids lutein and zeaxanthin, and/or omega-3 long-chain polyunsaturated fatty acids (ω-3 LCPUFAs) docosahexaenoic acid (DHA) and eicosapentaenoic acid (EPA) could further reduce the risk of AMD progression. AREDS 2 was also designed to investigate if eliminating beta carotene and/or lowering the dosage of zinc could be effective in preventing AMD progression [62].

All participants were randomly assigned to: (1) placebo (n = 1012); (2) L + Z (10 mg/2 mg, n = 1044); (3) ω-3 LCPUFAs (eicosapentaenoic acid (EPA) + docosahexaenoic acid (DHA) [650gmg/350 mg] n = 1069); or (4) the combination of L + Z and ω-3 LCPUFAs (n = 1078). All participants were offered a secondary randomization to 1 of 4 variations of the original AREDS formulation keeping vitamins C (500 mg), E (400 IU), and copper (2 mg) unchanged while varying zinc and beta-carotene as follows: zinc remains at the original level (80 mg), lower only zinc to 25 mg, omit beta-carotene only, or lower zinc to 25 mg and omit beta-carotene [62].

The results did not show a significant risk reduction with the addition of lutein and zeaxanthin or DHA and EPA. There was also no significant effect of the elimination of beta carotene or lowering the zinc dosage. Thus, it was determined that lutein and zeaxanthin could be an effective and safe substitute for beta carotene considering the higher association of lung cancer in current smokers or former smokers taking beta carotene. There is no reported association of lutein and zeaxanthin with lung cancer. It was determined the dosage of zinc could be lowered without any harmful adverse effects [62]. In conclusion, it is now recommended that patients with intermediate AMD or advanced disease in one eye (but not the other) should consider taking an AREDS 2-based supplement along with a broad-spectrum multivitamin to prevent the progression to advanced AMD.

The Rotterdam Study, a prospective, population-based study, investigated whether dietary nutrients and antioxidants reduce the incidence of developing early AMD in people aged 55 or older who are at a high genetic risk [63]. The study investigated the CFH Y402H and LOC387715 A69S gene variants which have been said to increase the risk of developing AMD if present. In the presence of the CFH Y402H gene and the LOC387715 A69S gene, the risk of AMD increases by 11 and 15 times, respectively [63]. This study sought to demonstrate any synergistic effects of CFH Y402H and LOC387715 A69S with nutrients [63].

The results showed a positive interaction of CFH Y402H with zinc, beta carotene, lutein, zeaxanthin, EPA, and DHA. In addition, there was a positive interaction of LOC387715 A69S with zinc, EPA, and DHA. The study determined that zinc, beta carotene, lutein, zeaxanthin, EPA, and DHA reduce the risk of developing early AMD in individuals who are considered to be at high genetic risk [63]. The authors recommended for this high genetic risk group to a diet rich in these nutrients. Foods rich in zinc include fortified cereals, meats, dairy products, nuts, and seeds. Foods rich in beta carotene, lutein and zeaxanthin include dark green leafy vegetables such as spinach and kale, egg yolk, and orange vegetables including carrots, peppers, and pumpkin. Foods rich in EPA and DHA include oily fish such as herring, salmon, sardines, trout, and tuna [63].

6. Discussion

Health promotion is a daunting concept due to the wide range of elements under its umbrella. One goal of health promotion is to empower the patient, giving them responsibility so that they are in charge of their own health care. Giving them the responsibility for their health will allow patients to set expectations and understand the consequences if not followed. The patient empowerment model ensures that health promotion is applied in the exam rather than occurring after the visit. Managing risks mirrors health promotion's overall goal. Patients at high risk for health complications need to be managed more closely and provided with the appropriate education to maximize their outcomes.

Patient-centered care is the foundation of health promotion, where the patient's treatment and management are actively tailored to best fit them, considering outside factors specific to the patient [11]. Communication is essential in maximizing the patient's outcome; however, it must be delivered effectively. Communicating with the patient should not be rushed or insensitive, especially when the patient's health is not optimal at that moment. Patients can become discouraged if they sense their health care provider is not invested in their care.

Communication can vary to include written, verbal or role modeling forms, depending on the case and patient. Up-to-date knowledge and skills are enforced in the field of nursing to give the patient the most appropriate treatments while upholding the health promotion model. Coordinated care is where multiple disciplines and/or professions can communicate with one another and keep each other updated on the current status of their patient. Patients with chronic illnesses typically have more than one provider for their care. By coordinating care with an inter-professional model, the patient's health care providers will be updated on the recent findings from the other providers caring for the patient. This communication is key to optimizing the flow, experience and care of the patient.

Health promotion can play a large role in educating patients on ways to reduce their risk of AMD, considering the modifiable risk factors involved in the disease. Getting the message across to the targeted audience depends largely on the accessibility of information. Health promotion can occur in schools, clinics, workplaces, residential areas and local community centers where people may gather and learn about how to take control of their health. Effective promotion addresses health while also taking into consideration the full spectrum of influences affecting health. For example, it considers cultural and social behaviors that are most prevalent in that particular setting. To properly deliver the information, there needs to be a strategic approach on how to convey the message for each specific population. Any disease can be addressed for each population if divided into the following four categories: healthy population, population with risk factors, population with symptoms, and population with the disease. Kumar et al., developed a flow chart that shows the categories and what topics need to be covered to effectively communicate the message [11].

For healthy populations, topics such as lifestyle and prevention of risk factors with primordial prevention need to be addressed. Primordial prevention is used to lessen the incidence of a disease by educating the individual before they become symptomatic. In this model, they are given the necessary knowledge and tools to reduce their risk considering their environmental, socioeconomic, behavioral conditions, and cultural practices [11]. For a population at risk, there must be active health promotion including how to overcome modifiable risk factors and attending regular appointments with members of the health care team. The population with symptoms specifically needs access to medical care for early detection, treatment and management, promotion of a healthy lifestyle.

If there is a disability resulting from the condition, rehabilitation will have an important role. The population with the known disorder must be offered treatment and care, healthy lifestyle reinforcement and any disability and rehabilitation services needed. Chronic diseases have grown to be a main factor in global mortality. Health promotion can be used for individuals with non-communicable diseases where an intervention can be initiated to avoid further progression. For example, health promotion alone can prevent heart disease and stroke by 80%, diabetes by 80% and 40% of cancers by reducing major risk factors that exacerbate their development [11].

AMD is a multifactorial disease where nutrition and diet play a significant role in potentially reducing the risk of its development and progression. With age, there is an increase in the production of free radicals, causing oxidative stress exacerbating the aging of tissues. A growing body of evidence suggests a key pathogenetic factor involves chronic inflammation and immunosenescence, which may be brought on by sustained oxidative stress paired with reduced antioxidant capacity [25, 32, 33, 40]. Given that systemic low-grade inflammation may be strongly influenced by the gut microbiota, particularly among older adults [64], sufficient absorption of these protective micronutrients is essential for promoting redox balance [65–67]. Antioxidants and other nutrients decrease the oxidative stress occurring in the eyes. Examples include vitamins (C, D, and E), zinc, and carotenoids (lutein and zeaxanthin) [40, 68]. Interestingly, these antioxidants work together by a protective chain where they assist each other when one is in the process of neutralizing free radicals. Vitamins C and E, along with lutein and zeaxanthin, arguably share a significant role in that antioxidant network.

The Mediterranean diet has been studied and recommended for its healthy foods which have shown show an association to lower mortality and cancer rates, and reduced risk of AMD [69]. Consequently, this type of diet decreases the amount of inflammation and oxidative stress in the body and ultimately in the retina.

The Mediterranean diet is rich in fruits, legumes, vegetables, bread, cereals, potatoes, beans, nuts, seeds, olive oil [69]. The diet includes low to moderate amounts of dairy products and alcohol with even lower quantities of red meats. This diet is in contrast to the typical pro-inflammatory Western diet. A report in The American Journal of Nutrition showed a 26% reduction in the progression to advanced AMD in participants who strictly adhered to a Mediterranean diet alone [69]. The study also showed that the addition of AREDS supplementation did not further decrease the risk when coupled with the Mediterranean diet. Overall, the study proved following this diet rich in fruits, vegetables and lean protein can aid in slowing the progression to advanced AMD [69].

In understanding the association of AMD, nutrition, and systemic factors, can motivate their patients to take control of their ocular health. Primary care physicians should recommend regular eye examinations including a dilated retinal examination to assess for AMD and other conditions. In addition, encourage patients to visit their eye care provider whenever the patient experiences a change in their vision. This gives the eye care providers a better chance to detect and manage early disease before extensive damage has occurred. Dry AMD is most associated with complaints of gradual decrease in vision while rapid vision loss is more closely associated with wet AMD.

All health care providers can educate their patients that unhealthy habits such as smoking can cause damage to their retina and ultimately their vision. At times, patients tend to not take their chronic illness seriously because they may not see any obvious physical signs. To emphasize the importance of controlling their chronic illness, the primary care provider can warn the patient that their unhealthy choices can consequently lead to irreversible vision loss. It is possible the patient may become more concerned when it is brought to their attention that their vision could be irreversibly damaged.

If health promotion is effectively initiated and maintained, the patient may be more willing to take control of their condition, improve their adherence to treatments, maintain their follow-up appointments, and self-monitor their illnesses.

Conflict of interest

Alexander Martinez None Joseph Pizzimenti None Drake W. Lem none. Dr. Pinakin Gunvant Davey none.

Author details

Alexander Martinez[1,2], Joseph J. Pizzimenti[1], Drake W. Lem[3]
and Pinakin Gunvant Davey[3*]

1 Rosenberg School of Optometry, University of Incarnate Word,
San Antonio Texas USA

2 South Texas Eye Institute, San Antonio, Texas, USA

3 College of Optometry, Western University of Health Sciences, Pomona California
USA

*Address all correspondence to: contact@pinakindavey.com

IntechOpen

References

[1] Schwartz R, Loewenstein A. Early detection of age related macular degeneration: Current status. International Journal of Retina and Vitreous. 2015;**1**(1):20

[2] Spaide RF, Jaffe GJ, Sarraf D, Freund KB, Sadda SR, Staurenghi G, et al. Consensus nomenclature for reporting neovascular age-related macular degeneration data: Consensus on neovascular age-related macular degeneration nomenclature study group. Ophthalmology. 2020;**127**(5): 616-636

[3] Pennington KL, DeAngelis MM. Epidemiology of age-related macular degeneration (AMD): Associations with cardiovascular disease phenotypes and lipid factors. Eye and Vision (London). 2016;**3**(1):34

[4] Zhang QY, Tie LJ, Wu SS, Lv PL, Huang HW, Wang WQ, et al. Overweight, obesity, and risk of age-related macular degeneration. Investigative Ophthalmology & Visual Science. 2016;**57**(3):1276-1283

[5] Ho L, van Leeuwen R, de Jong PTVM, Vingerling JR, Klaver CCW. Epidemiology of AMD. Age-related Macular Degeneration. Second ed2013. pp. 3-32

[6] Garcia-Layana A, Cabrera-Lopez F, Garcia-Arumi J, Arias-Barquet L, Ruiz-Moreno JM. Early and intermediate age-related macular degeneration: Update and clinical review. Clinical Interventions in Aging. 2017;**12**:1579-1587

[7] Meyers KJ, Liu Z, Millen AE, Iyengar SK, Blodi BA, Johnson E, et al. Joint associations of diet, lifestyle, and genes with age-related macular degeneration. Ophthalmology. 2015;**122**(11):2286-2294

[8] Bourne RRA, Jonas JB, Bron AM, Cicinelli MV, Das A, Flaxman SR, et al. Prevalence and causes of vision loss in high-income countries and in eastern and Central Europe in 2015: Magnitude, temporal trends and projections. The British Journal of Ophthalmology. 2018;**102**(5):575-585

[9] National Eye Institute. Age-Related Macular Degeneration 2021 [updated 2020/08/17]. Available from: https://www.nei.nih.gov/learn-about-eye-health/eye-conditions-and-diseases/age-related-macular-degeneration

[10] Jager RD, Mieler WF, Miller JW. Age-related macular degeneration. The New England Journal of Medicine. 2008;**358**(24):2606-2617

[11] Kumar S, Preetha G. Health promotion: An effective tool for global health. Indian Journal of Community Medicine. 2012;**37**(1):5-12

[12] Mathenge W. Age-related macular degeneration. Community Eye Health. 2014;**27**(87):49-50

[13] Age-Related Eye Disease Study Research G. Risk factors associated with age-related macular degeneration. A case-control study in the age-related eye disease study: Age-Related Eye Disease Study Report Number 3. Ophthalmology. 2000;**107**(12): 2224-2232

[14] Ferris FL 3rd, Wilkinson CP, Bird A, Chakravarthy U, Chew E, Csaky K, et al. Clinical classification of age-related macular degeneration. Ophthalmology. 2013;**120**(4):844-851

[15] Dietzel M, Pauleikhoff D, Holz FG, AC BI. Early AMD. Age-related Macular Degeneration. Second ed2013. pp. 100-109

[16] Ambati J, Fowler BJ. Mechanisms of age-related macular degeneration. Neuron. 2012;**75**(1):26-39

[17] Owsley C, McGwin G Jr, Clark ME, Jackson GR, Callahan MA, Kline LB, et al. Delayed rod-mediated dark adaptation is a functional biomarker for incident early age-related macular degeneration. Ophthalmology. 2016;**123**(2):344-351

[18] Spaide RF. Clinical Manifestations of Choroidal Neovascularization in AMD. Age-related Macular Degeneration. Second ed2013. pp. 110-119

[19] Fleckenstein M, Schmitz-Valckenberg S, Sunness JS, Holz FG. Geographic Atrophy. Age-related Macular Degeneration. Second ed2013. pp. 120-138

[20] Velilla S, Garcia-Medina JJ, Garcia-Layana A, Dolz-Marco R, Pons-Vazquez S, Pinazo-Duran MD, et al. Smoking and age-related macular degeneration: Review and update. Journal of Ophthalmology. 2013; **2013**:895147

[21] Caban-Martinez AJ, Davila EP, Lam BL, Dubovy SR, McCollister KE, Fleming LE, et al. Age-related macular degeneration and smoking cessation advice by eye care providers: a pilot study. Preventing Chronic Disease. 2011;**8**(6):A147-A

[22] Choudhury F, Varma R, McKean-Cowdin R, Klein R, Azen SP. Risk factors for four-year incidence and progression of age-related macular degeneration: The Los Angeles Latino eye study. American Journal of Ophthalmology. 2011;**152**(3):385-395

[23] Lambert NG, ElShelmani H, Singh MK, Mansergh FC, Wride MA, Padilla M, et al. Risk factors and biomarkers of age-related macular degeneration. Progress in Retinal and Eye Research. 2016;**54**:64-102

[24] Klein R, Klein BE, Tomany SC, Moss SE. Ten-year incidence of age-related maculopathy and smoking and drinking: The beaver dam eye study. American Journal of Epidemiology. 2002;**156**(7):589-598

[25] Bernstein PS, Li B, Vachali PP, Gorusupudi A, Shyam R, Henriksen BS, et al. Lutein, zeaxanthin, and meso-zeaxanthin: The basic and clinical science underlying carotenoid-based nutritional interventions against ocular disease. Progress in Retinal and Eye Research. 2016;**50**:34-66

[26] Davey PG, Alvarez SD, Lee JY. Macular pigment optical density: Repeatability, intereye correlation, and effect of ocular dominance. Clinical Ophthalmology. 2016;**10**:1671-1678

[27] Davey PG, Ngo A, Cross J, Gierhart DL. Macular Pigment Reflectometry: Development and Evaluation of a Novel Clinical Device for Rapid Objective Assessment of the Macular Carotenoids. In: Manns F, Soderberg PG, Ho a, Editors. Ophthalmic Technologies Xxix. Proceedings of SPIE. 10858. Bellingham: Spie-Int Soc Optical Engineering; 2019

[28] Davey PG, Rosen RB, Gierhart DL. Macular pigment reflectometry: Developing clinical protocols, comparison with heterochromatic flicker photometry and individual carotenoid levels. Nutrients. 2021;**13**(8):2553

[29] Howells O, Eperjesi F, Bartlett H. Measuring macular pigment optical density in vivo: A review of techniques. Graefe's Archive for Clinical and Experimental Ophthalmology. 2011;**249**(3):315-347

[30] Leung IY. Macular pigment: New clinical methods of detection and the role of carotenoids in age-related macular degeneration. Optometry. 2008;**79**(5):266-272

[31] Yung M, Klufas MA, Sarraf D. Clinical applications of fundus

autofluorescence in retinal disease. International Journal of Retina and Vitreous. 2016;**2**:12

[32] Lem DW, Gierhart DL, Davey PG. Management of Diabetic Eye Disease using Carotenoids and Nutrients. Antioxidants - Benefits, Sources, and Mechanisms of Action. London: IntechOpen; 2021

[33] Lem DW, Gierhart DL, Davey PG. A systematic review of carotenoids in the management of diabetic retinopathy. Nutrients. 2021;**13**(7):2441

[34] Boulton ME. Ageing of the Retina and Retinal Pigment Epithelium. Age-related Macular Degeneration. Second ed2013. pp. 45-59

[35] Deangelis MM, Silveira AC, Carr EA, Kim IK. Genetics of age-related macular degeneration: Current concepts, future directions. Seminars in Ophthalmology. 2011;**26**(3):77-93

[36] Turbert D. What Is Optical Coherence Tomography? 2020. Available from: https://www.aao.org/eye-health/treatments/what-is-optical-coherence-tomography

[37] Porter D, Turbert D. What Is Fluorescein Angiography? 2018. Available from: https://www.aao.org/eye-health/treatments/what-is-fluorescein-angiography

[38] Ma L, Dou HL, Huang YM, Lu XR, Xu XR, Qian F, et al. Improvement of retinal function in early age-related macular degeneration after lutein and zeaxanthin supplementation: A randomized, double-masked, placebo-controlled trial. American Journal of Ophthalmology. 2012;**154**(4): 625-634 e1

[39] Johnson EJ, Avendano EE, Mohn ES, Raman G. The association between macular pigment optical density and visual function outcomes: A systematic review and meta-analysis. Eye (London, England). 2020

[40] Lem DW, Davey PG, Gierhart DL, Rosen RB. A systematic review of carotenoids in the management of age-related macular degeneration. Antioxidants (Basel). 2021;**10**(8):1255

[41] Liu R, Wang T, Zhang B, Qin L, Wu C, Li Q, et al. Lutein and zeaxanthin supplementation and association with visual function in age-related macular degeneration. Investigative Ophthalmology & Visual Science. 2014;**56**(1):252-258

[42] Ma L, Liu R, Du JH, Liu T, Wu SS, Liu XH. Lutein, zeaxanthin and Meso-zeaxanthin supplementation associated with macular pigment optical density. Nutrients. 2016;**8**(7):426

[43] Huang YM, Dou HL, Huang FF, Xu XR, Zou ZY, Lin XM. Effect of supplemental lutein and zeaxanthin on serum, macular pigmentation, and visual performance in patients with early age-related macular degeneration. BioMed Research International. 2015;**2015**:564738

[44] Meleth AD, Raiji VR, Krishnadev N, Chew EY. Nutritional Supplementation in AMD. Age-related Macular Degeneration. Second ed2013. pp. 191-202

[45] Seddon JM. Macular degeneration epidemiology: Nature-nurture, lifestyle factors, genetic risk, and gene-environment interactions - the Weisenfeld award lecture. Investigative Ophthalmology & Visual Science. 2017;**58**(14):6513-6528

[46] Tripathy K, Salini B. Amsler Grid. StatPearls. Treasure Island (FL): StatPearls Publishing; 2020

[47] Age-Related Eye Disease Study Research G. A randomized, placebo-controlled, clinical trial of high-dose

supplementation with vitamins C and E, beta carotene, and zinc for age-related macular degeneration and vision loss: AREDS report no. 8. Archives of Ophthalmology. 2001;**119**(10):1417-1436

[48] Duffy AM, Bouchier-Hayes DJ, Harmey JH. Vascular Endothelial Growth Factor (VEGF) and its Role in Non-Endothelial Cells: Autocrine Signalling by VEGF. Madame Curie Bioscience Database [Internet]. Landes Bioscience: Austin (TX); 2000-2013

[49] Kim LA, D'Amore PA. A brief history of anti-VEGF for the treatment of ocular angiogenesis. The American Journal of Pathology. 2012;**181**(2): 376-379

[50] Schmidt-Erfurth U, Chong V, Loewenstein A, Larsen M, Souied E, Schlingemann R, et al. Guidelines for the management of neovascular age-related macular degeneration by the European Society of Retina Specialists (EURETINA). The British Journal of Ophthalmology. 2014;**98**(9):1144-1167

[51] WHO. WHO Health Promotion. 2016. Available from: https://www.who.int/news-room/questions-and-answers/item/health-promotion

[52] Jandorf S, Krogh Nielsen M, Sorensen K, Sorensen TL. Low health literacy levels in patients with chronic retinal disease. BMC Ophthalmology. 2019;**19**(1):174

[53] McGuinness MB, Le J, Mitchell P, Gopinath B, Cerin E, Saksens NTM, et al. Physical activity and age-related macular degeneration: A systematic literature review and meta-analysis. American Journal of Ophthalmology. 2017;**180**:29-38

[54] Berrow EJ, Bartlett HE, Eperjesi F, Gibson JM. The effects of a lutein-based supplement on objective and subjective measures of retinal and visual function in eyes with age-related maculopathy—a randomised controlled trial. The British Journal of Nutrition. 2013;**109**(11): 2008-2014

[55] Huang YM, Dou HL, Huang FF, Xu XR, Zou ZY, Lu XR, et al. Changes following supplementation with lutein and zeaxanthin in retinal function in eyes with early age-related macular degeneration: A randomised, double-blind, placebo-controlled trial. The British Journal of Ophthalmology. 2015;**99**(3):371-375

[56] Seddon JM, Cote J, Davis N, Rosner B. Progression of age-related macular degeneration: Association with body mass index, waist circumference, and waist-hip ratio. Archives of Ophthalmology. 2003;**121**(6):785-792

[57] Khoo HE, Ng HS, Yap WS, Goh HJH, Yim HS. Nutrients for prevention of macular degeneration and eye-related diseases. Antioxidants (Basel). 2019;**8**(4):85

[58] Shyam R, Gorusupudi A, Nelson K, Horvath MP, Bernstein PS. RPE65 has an additional function as the lutein to meso-zeaxanthin isomerase in the vertebrate eye. Proceedings of the National Academy of Sciences of the United States of America. 2017; **114**(41):10882-10887

[59] Davey PG, Henderson T, Lem DW, Weis R, Amonoo-Monney S, Evans DW. Visual function and macular carotenoid changes in eyes with retinal drusen-an open label randomized controlled trial to compare a micronized lipid-based carotenoid liquid supplementation and AREDS-2 formula. Nutrients. 2020;**12**(11):1-12

[60] Bone RA, Davey PG, Roman BO, Evans DW. Efficacy of commercially available nutritional supplements: Analysis of serum uptake, macular pigment optical density and visual functional response. Nutrients. 2020;**12**(5):15

[61] Age-Related Eye Disease Study Research G. The Age-Related Eye Disease Study (AREDS): design implications. AREDS report no. 1. Controlled Clinical Trials. 1999;**20**(6): 573-600

[62] Age-Related Eye Disease Study 2 Research G, Chew EY, Clemons TE, JP SG, Danis R, Ferris FL, et al. Lutein + zeaxanthin and omega-3 fatty acids for age-related macular degeneration: the Age-Related Eye Disease Study 2 (AREDS2) randomized clinical trial. JAMA. 2013;**309**(19):2005-2015

[63] Ho L, van Leeuwen R, Witteman JC, van Duijn CM, Uitterlinden AG, Hofman A, et al. Reducing the genetic risk of age-related macular degeneration with dietary antioxidants, zinc, and omega-3 fatty acids: The Rotterdam study. Archives of Ophthalmology. 2011;**129**(6):758-766

[64] Ticinesi A, Lauretani F, Milani C, Nouvenne A, Tana C, Del Rio D, et al. Aging gut microbiota at the Cross-road between nutrition, physical frailty, and sarcopenia: Is there a gut-muscle Axis? Nutrients. 2017;**9**(12):1303

[65] Andriessen EM, Wilson AM, Mawambo G, Dejda A, Miloudi K, Sennlaub F, et al. Gut microbiota influences pathological angiogenesis in obesity-driven choroidal neovascularization. EMBO Molecular Medicine. 2016;**8**(12):1366-1379

[66] Lima-Fontes M, Meira L, Barata P, Falcao M, Carneiro A. Gut microbiota and age-related macular degeneration: A growing partnership. Survey of Ophthalmology. 2021, 6257;(21):00213

[67] Rinninella E, Mele MC, Merendino N, Cintoni M, Anselmi G, Caporossi A, et al. The role of diet, micronutrients and the gut microbiota in age-related macular degeneration: New perspectives from the gut(−)retina Axis. Nutrients. 2018;**10**(11):1677

[68] Carneiro A, Andrade JP. Nutritional and lifestyle interventions for age-related macular degeneration: A review. Oxidative Medicine and Cellular Longevity. 2017;**2017**:6469138

[69] Merle BM, Silver RE, Rosner B, Seddon JM. Adherence to a Mediterranean diet, genetic susceptibility, and progression to advanced macular degeneration: A prospective cohort study. The American Journal of Clinical Nutrition. 2015;**102**(5):1196-1206

Section 3

Treatment

Chapter 4

Anti-VEGF Treatment and Optical Coherence Tomography Biomarkers in Wet Age-Related Macular Degeneration

Maja Vinković, Andrijana Kopić and Tvrtka Benašić

Abstract

Age-related macular degeneration (AMD) is one of the most common causes of severe visual loss in middle and old-age population, and often leads to serious deterioration in quality of life. Currently, the first-line treatment for neovascular AMD (nAMD) are intravitreal injections of anti-vascular endothelial growth factor (VEGF) medications, including bevacizumab, ranibizumab, and aflibercept and also latest commercially available drug, brolucizumab. During initial examination and imaging and treatment follow-up for patients with nAMD, optical coherence tomography (OCT) is used to predict and assess the therapeutic response and guide the treatment. Several OCT-based biomarkers, including the central subfoveal thickness (CSFT), the presence of intraretinal cysts (IRCs) or subretinal fluid (SRF), and the presence of pigment epithelial detachment (PED), were found to influence baseline visual acuity or visual improvements. Recent analyses of large randomized control trials (RCTs) summarized the usefulness of these OCT-based biomarkers. However, many of these early studies relied on time-domain OCT to evaluate the retinal structures thus providing less precise evaluation of the retinal details. After introduction of spectral-domain OCT (SD-OCT) which provided high resolution images, recent studies offered new insights in specific morphological changes and their different impact on visual function in nAMD. For example, these advancement in resolution offered new classification of IRCs into degenerative and exudative which impacts treatment strategy and final outcome in the treatment of nAMD. Moreover, the recent data disclose a substantial difference between RCTs and real-world studies regarding the response to anti-VEGF therapy. In conclusions, IRCs and PED are associated with poor visual improvement in nAMD in a realworld setting. Both IRCs and SRF responded better than PED to anti-VEGF therapy. These observations mandate large longitudinal studies focusing on the usefulness of these high resolution SD-OCT biomarkers in real-world situations.

Keywords: Anti-VEGF treatment, biomarkers, intraretinal cysts, intraretinal fluid, neovascular AMD, OCT, pigment epithelial detachment, subretinal fluid

1. Introduction

Improving or maintaining visual acuity is the main target of treatment of neo-vascular age-related macular degeneration (nAMD). Standard nAMD care mandate frequent intravitreal (IVT) antivascular endothelial growth factor (VEGF) injections, which represents a heavy burden on patients, health systems, and physicians.

Age-related macular degeneration (AMD) is the leading cause of blindness in developed countries, with a global prevalence of 8.69% [1]. The prevalence of AMD increases with age among all ethnicities and in all geographic regions, as a result of a growing aging population [2].

Age-related macular degeneration is a progressive, chronic, multifactorial disease of the retina that can lead to visual impairment and blindness, mostly affecting individuals aged more than 60 years [3]. The disease progresses from early to advanced stages and can be divided into 2 major advanced forms: neovascular (wet) AMD (nAMD) and geographic atrophy in dry AMD [4]. A smaller proportion of patients with AMD (20%) are diagnosed with nAMD, but it is responsible for the majority (90%) of vision loss cases and presents as acute painless loss of vision [5, 6]. Neovascular AMD is characterized by the presence of choroidal neovascularization (CNV), a pathologic form of angiogenesis resulting in leakage of fluid that accumulates in the retina, subretinally or below the retinal pigment epithelium (RPE); other features include the development of RPE tears, hard exudates, hemorrhage, or fibrous disciform scar tissue formation [7–9].

These clinical abnormalities in patients with nAMD lead to a gradual loss of retinal photoreceptors, resulting in decreased vision and even blindness if disease progression is not prevented [10].

Central vision is the key to variuos daily activities, including a person's ability to read, drive, and recognize faces [11]. The loss of central vision that accompanies AMD greatly affects an individual's quality of life [12].

Deleterious effect of vision loss on an individual's quality of life mandates further development of effective treatment modalities and new molecules to treat nAMD.

2. Advances in nAMD treatment

Preservation of visual function is the main goal for nAMD treatment. This is achieved by inhibition of the new blood vessel growth and reduction of the fluid leakage [13]. Vascular endothelial growth factor is a major molecule which contributes to development of CNV [14]. Choroidal neovascularization can be slowed by inhibiting VEGF binding to its receptor, VEGF receptor-2, on blood vessels, which is the major proangiogenic pathway [15]. Anti-VEGF agents are antibodies which neutralize VEGF binding to its receptor and they have different mechanisms of action. They reduce fluid leakage from the CNV, stop growth, and lead to regression of CNV [16]. The introduction of the anti-VEGF drugs into clinical practice has immensely improved the prognosis for patients with nAMD, in such a way that nAMD is no longer considered an incurable disease [17]. The first anti-VEGF agent approved in 2004 by Food and Drug Administration (FDA) was pegaptanib sodium, an aptamer that binds $VEGF_{165}$ [18]. Ranibizumab, an antibody fragment that binds all VEGF-A isoforms was FDA approved in 2006 after the ANCHOR and MARINA studies [19, 20]. In the following years, from 2006 till 2013, there were 2 other anti-VEGF therapies available for nAMD treatment: aflibercept and conbercept, approved based on the results of the VIEW 1 and VIEW 2 studies, and PHOENIX study, respectively [21, 22]. Both of them are antibody fusion proteins [23].

Two other anti-VEGF agents approved for therapy in oncology are used "off-label" for nAMD: ziv-aflibercept and bevacizumab [7]. Current care standards for nAMD include regular intravitreal (IVT) injections of anti-VEGF therapy [24]. This poses a substantial burden on patients, as well as health systems worldwide [3]. For some patients, anti-VEGF treatment involves monthly injections over a long period of time, making patient adherence and monitoring difficult, which in turn has consequences for visual and anatomic outcomes [25]. Also, the cost associated with managing nAMD is substantial [26]. In an attempt to lessen the load of frequent therapy and costs associated with anti-VEGF medications, some clinicians proposed alternative dosing strategies which are different from those in the registered clinical trials (q4- or q8-weeks). These include pro re nata (PRN) and treat-and-extend (TAE) regimens [27]. They attempt to provide the same efficacy and at the same time more convenient regimen that is easier to adhere to and is taking into account individual OCT features of the patient.

Brolucizumab, a newly developed anti-VEGF drug for nAMD treatment, has demonstrated longer durability and improvement in visual and anatomic outcomes in clinical studies in a q12-week regimen, indicating its potential to reduce treatment burden as an important therapeutic tool in nAMD management [28].

3. The role of OCT + OCT-A in nAMD

3.1 Specific OCT biomarkers

Several OCT-based biomarkers, including the central subfoveal thickness (CSFT), the presence of intraretinal cysts (IRCs) or fluid (IRF), subretinal fluid (SRF), and sub-RPE fluid or pigment epithelial detachment (PED), were found to be associated with baseline visual acuity and response to the anti-VEGF treatment (**Figure 1**). One of the main goals in the management of nAMD has been the removal of fluid in the macular compartments [26]. The clinical significance of fluid depends on its location where it plays a major role in determining the long term success of the treatment and its presence should be recorded at baseline, according to the guidelines from the Vision Academy. Fluid segments should be assesed individually and fluid status evaluated after loading phase and throughout the course of treatment [29, 30].

The introduction of OCT into everyday clinical practice allowed a new classification of CNV according to its location, complementing fluorescein angiography (FA) and indocyanin green angiography (ICGA) [31]. In OCT, type 1 CNV, located between Bruch membrane (BM) and RPE, corresponds to PED, often accompanied

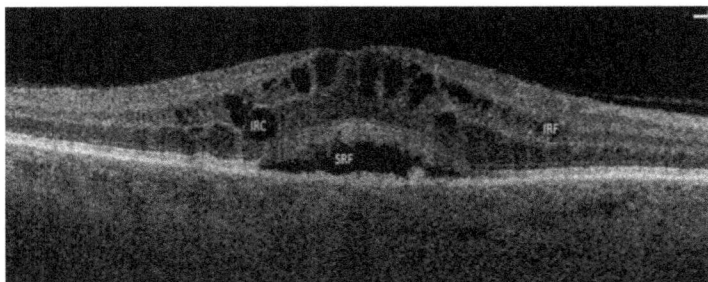

Figure 1.
OCT biomarkers.

by subretinal fluid and in later stages of disease by IRC [32]. Type 2 CNV presents as subretinal hyperreflective material (SHRM) and shows concomitant IRF and SRF [33]. SHRM may be composed of exudative fluid, fibrin, blood, or scarring and its characteristics may change during treatment period [34]. According to CATT study, SHRM was present in 77% of treatment-naive eyes at baseline with the prevalence decreasing to 58% at week 4 after treatment and further to 46% after 2 years [35]. It is hypothesized to be caused probably by a dehydration and condensation of the active CNV component [36, 37].

IRC overlying PED, accompanied by SRF, are typical features commonly present in retinal angiomatous proliferation (RAP), classified as type 3 CNV by Freund et al. [38]. Mature type 3 lesions, associated with serous PEDs, are highly responsive to anti-VEGF therapy [39]. However, the development of GA has frequently been described in association with treatment of RAP lesions [40].

3.1.1 Central subfoveal thickness

The greatest importance of CSFT was actually in the research because it was used as a criterion for continued treatment in trials of various drugs and treatment protocols. If the reduction in CSFT after injection is less than 25%, this is considered a criterion for reinjection [41, 42].

Value of CSFT depends mostly on the amount of retinal fluid in the different retinal compartments, so in most cases a higher CSFT is also a sign of a worse VA. If the cause of CSFT is mostly retinal fluid, it will be reduced by treatment with anti-VEGF factors, and VA in this case will be better or not get worse. Recently there was an observation that there is a direct correlation between vision, fluid, the amount of fluid, and fluctuations in CST [28]. A new option is to look at what effect a drug has on fluctuations in CST, which may prove to be extremely important in identifying patients at risk for closer monitoring and more aggressive therapy.

The presence of an epiretinal membrane (ERM) and the accumulation of drusenoid or fibrous material may also be responsible for a higher CSFT. In this case, the prognosis for CSFT reduction with anti-VEGF treatment is usually poor [28, 41].

A certain percentage of subjects in clinical trials as well as patients in clinical practice developed geographic atrophy (GA) after treatment with anti-VEGF factors. Risk factors for such development include the presence of foveal fluid and monthly dosing of injections. In the CATT study, approximately 38% of subjects developed GA after 5 years, mainly those receiving ranibizumab rather than aflibercept. In the case of GA development, a lower CSFT will also mean a significantly lower VA [7, 43].

3.1.2 Intraretinal fluid

Intraretinal fluid appears as round or oval hyporeflective spaces – cysts, but may also present as diffuse thickening of the neurosensory retina [1]. Intraretinal cysts (IRCs) are OCT biomarkers for various retinal diseases such as nAMD, diabetic macular edema, central retinal vein occlusion, and uveitic macular edema.

Since IRCs often differ in their shape and size, and also in their response to anti-VEGF therapy, some authors have divided them into exudative and degenerative. The criteria taken into account were the size of the cyst, its shape, and the possible alteration of the continuity of the RPE below the cyst. Degenerative cysts were described as smaller than 125 μm, usually square in shape and with RPE alterations below the cyst itself, while exudative cysts are more often ovoid and larger [41, 44, 45]. Intraretinal fluid usually results from active fluid exudation, but the degenerative cysts may orginate from passive fluid accumulation due to atrophy of neurosensory elements [1]. Exudative cysts had better initial response to 3 loading monthly injections of anti-VEGF treatment whereas degenerative cysts had lower response to the therapy, persisted for a longer time and were associated with lower VA after treatment [44–47].

3.1.3 Subretinal fluid

Subretinal fluid can be characterized as hyporeflective fluid accumulation overlying the RPE layer. It resolves in most eyes in response to anti-VEGF treatment, however, not as rapidly as IRF.

According to the several studies, the presence of SRF at baseline or after 1-year treatment did not significantly affect VA [44, 48, 49]. Residual SRF may not always represent ongoing neovascular activity. It may instead be dysfunction of the RPE leading to SRF accumulation, much like central serous chorioretinopathy [50, 51]. Among patients treated with a PRN regimen, those who presented with SRF achieved even higher VA gains [52]. VA was stable regardless of treatment frequency [53]. The pathomechanism for the beneficial role of SRF has not been fully explained but possible explanations suggest the preservation of photoreceptor integrity, less IRF, RPE atrophy and fibrosis [54].

3.1.4 Pigment epithelial detachment

Pigment epithelial detachment (PED) (**Figure 2**) the anatomical separation of the RPE from the Bruch membrane i.e. sub-RPE fluid is present in about 30–80% of nAMD patients based on the CATT, EXCITE, and VIEW studies [41, 55, 56].

PED lesions have been classified based on clinical findings, angiography and OCT assessment (height, width, greatest linear diameter, area, volume, reflectivity, progression and response to treatment of PED lesions) [57]. Three subtypes of PED may be identified based on the reflectivity of the material under the RPE: serous (primarily hyporeflective; hollow), solid (primarily hyperreflective; drusenoid), and mixed (combination of solid and serous PEDs; fibrovascular) [58–60]. The CNV membrane itself corresponds to hyperreflective material along the back surface of the PED, readily visible by enhanced-depth imaging, or a tomographic notch within the PED, identifiable by conventional OCT [61].

PED has a negative effect on VA only in combination with additional components, mostly IRF [47, 62]. In VIEW studies, the baseline presence of PED, disrupted external limiting membrane (ELM) and ellipsoid zone (EZ), and greater CSFT were associated with poor baseline VA [46]. However there are some controversial data by real-world study where initial VA was worse and visual improvement

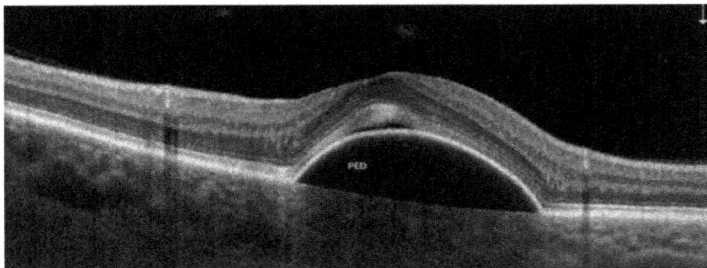

Figure 2.
Pigment epithelial detachment.

poorer if PED was present before treatment regardless of IRC or SRF presence [44]. Microperimetry analysis has shown higher retinal sensitivity for SRF and serous PED (sPED) than for IRF and fibrovascular PED (fvPED) [63]. The volume of fvPED at baseline was associated with impaired VA and PED growth seemed to precede fluid recurrence [64–66].

When SRF is located on the top of a PED (rather than on its edge), without associated IRF, hemorrhage, then probably the PED is not vascularized and will response poorly to anti-VEGF therapy [67]. PEDs are also less responsive to anti-VEGF treatment than SRF or IRC in nAMD [41, 46]. Serous PEDs showed better response to IVIs than fibrovascular ones which may suggest that they are possible signs of lesion activity. Serous PEDs showed most improvement in VA whereas fvPEDs showed most reduction in PED height, especially with aflibercept [50, 57, 68–70]. Fibrovascular PEDs may be difficult to treat, but even these eyes can gain vision with anti-VEGF therapy. The IVIs change PED morphology in such way that their content becomes more hyperreflective, suggesting an increasing fibrovascular maturization of the CNV [71]. PEDs behavior and functional outcomes are influenced by the treatment regimen. VIEW trials found that the switch from a monthly to an as-needed regimen led to reactivation of PED with a resultant decline in visual outcome, especially in patients who developed secondary IRC following that change [46]. The recurrence of PED is the primary event of neovascular activation [47].

Treatment should focus on vision gains rather than PED resolution because there is no apparent correlation between anatomical and functional improvement in most eyes with PED and nAMD. More frequent anti-VEGF doses may improve anatomical response, without correlation with vision improvement [29]. Atrophy may complicate eyes with PED and nAMD after anti-VEGF therapy, especially in association with complete PED resolution [29].

In 15–20% of eyes with PEDs a RPE tear that may lead to decline or loss of vision spontaneously but also as a serious complication of anti-VEGF therapy. Hyperreflective lines in near-infrared (NIR) images and PEDs greater than 500 μm to 600 μm in height on OCT present an indicator of an increased risk in developing an RPE tear in eyes where the sub-RPE CNV has created contractile folds in response to the treatment [72, 73]. RPE tears after anti-VEGF therapy only developed in patients with serous PED (14.6%) [74].

In conclusion, the presence or persistence of a PED may still be compatible with relatively good visual acuity, but may require more regular treatment.

3.2 Specific OCT-A biomarkers

Noninvasive OCT angiography (OCT-A) generates images of the retinal and choroidal vessels, with the excellent sensibility and specificity for detection of the CNV compared to FA and ICGA [75, 76]. OCT-A provides detailed visualization of the CNV complex in patients with nAMD and its evolution in response to anti-VEGF treatment, disclose a perfused vascular network in nonexudative stage of CNV and also in advanced cases of evident nAMD with fibrotic scars and history of prior treatment with anti-VEGF therapies [77]. CNV type 1 and 2 seem to be more easily visualised on OCT-A compared with retinal angiomatous proliferation (RAP) or polypoidal lesions [78].

Current studies evaluate the association between OCT-A parameters, structural OCT changes and functional response on anti-VEGF therapies. Five qualitative criteria have been recognized on OCT-A: (1) Numerous branching capillaries between major vessels separating the lesion area into fractals, (2) end-to-end anastomoses or intervascular anastomoses within the lesion, (3) arcades or vascular loops at the vessel termini, (4) major, well-defined filamentous vessels, and (5) peri- or intralesional nonvascularized hypointense halos surrounding or embedding the CNV membrane [75]. Greater rate of small branching vessels and peripheral arcades have been detected in immature lesions and a dead-tree appearance in hypermature lesions [79]. A qualitative classification algorithm has been developed based on neovascular density as a predictive factor for clinical activity [80]. Recently, some authors have demonstrated quantitative biomarkers for nAMD disease activity: (1) CNV's blood flow surface area (SA), (2) vessel density (VD), (3) fractal dimension (FD), and (4) lacunarity index (LAC) [81].

Blood flow SA is a readily available and well-studied OCT-A parameter. Previous qualitative assessments of OCT-A images in CNV networks showed that most of the lesions demonstrated shrinkage of fine peripheral vessels and arteriogenesis of the remaining vessels after anti-VEGF treatment [82]. The branching complexity and blood flow area decrease after the loading doses then regrow and return to the original size at 12 months irrespective of the treatment protocol. The same modifications of blood flow area in patients followed under PRN and TAE regimens [83]. SA also seems to have a weak association with functional outcomes (i.e. VA), highlighting the need to assess other parameters. Finally, the baseline blood flow area had an inverse association with the number of IVIs concerning baseline FD [83].

FD quantifies branching pattern complexity and organization of the vascular structure. It varies according to the number of secondary divisions of the CNV: the higher the number of discernible secondary divisions, the higher the FD value [84]. Many authors demonstrated attenuation and pruning of secondary ramifications after anti-VEGF treatments, with subsequent decrease of the FD value. A FD values is lower in the inactive stage than in the active stage [83, 84]. A weak association between blood flow aspect (FD) and retinal fluid suggests that factors other than CNV morphology are responsible for retinal exudation [79]. There is a poor association between the most studied quantitative OCT-A parameters and functional outcomes at 12 months' follow-up. FD did not differ between good and bad responders [83].

Lacunarity (LAC) is a measure of the size of gaps within a structure. Higher values reflect heterogenic texture of vascular networks and lower values reflect a more homogeneity of vascular skeleton. The results showed that arrangement of lacunas of the vascular plexus do not change after anti-VEGF, therefore lacunarity may be an OCT-A parameter for nAMD follow-up [85].

According to some investigators, patients with a lower baseline FD and a lower SA have higher odds of having 8 or more IVI injection during the first year. Typical examples of patients that required less than 8 IVI in the first year of treatment are large and complex CNVs. On the other hand, typical examples of patients that required more than eight IVI in the first year of treatments are small lesions with a disorganized architecture [83]. A hypothesis is that in the presence of high VEGF levels, CNVs would have numerous tiny branches and a disorganized architecture, reflecting an aggressive angiogenic process with greater exudation and a heavier treatment burden. In eyes with lower VEGF availability, CNV would grow without leakage maturing their branching architecture toward a complicated network before exudation becomes overly symptomatic [86]. In conclusion, it seems that all evaluated OCT-A parameters were poor biomarkers in predicting anatomic and functional response but baseline FD and SA were the best biomarkers regarding treatment burden.

4. The role of visual acuity on long term prognosis

Early response to anti-VEGF therapy has been shown to be an important predictor of VA recovery in nAMD treatment. VA after 3 months of consecutive intravitreal injections is a better prognostic factor than baseline VA [87]. Likewise, early morphological change of the described OCT biomarkers is a very important prognostic factor for overall treatment outcome.

Thus, early accurate monitoring of treatment responses by analysis of OCT findings and VA is of great importance to optimize the number of injections during treatment in achieving the goal of vision function recovery.

5. Conclusions

Introduction of OCT into everyday clinical practice has revolutionized diagnosis and management of nAMD. This diagnostic tool has pivotal role in terms of disease monitoring and evaluation of treatment efficacy. Many studies give hope that in the future we will be able to offer a better or possibly individual approach to the anti-VEGF treatment that will give the optimal morphological recovery of the macula and VA. The risk factors identified for persistent CNV activity may help clinicians to identify patients for closer monitoring and more aggressive therapy.

The main OCT features predictive of persistent disease activity are IRCs, SRF, sPED recurrence, and those indicative of poorer VA outcome are IRCs, large extent of SHRM damage to the photoreceptor or RPE layer [35]. Exudative IRCs have been shown to require monthly treatment, in particular after recurrence of PED [37, 88]. Patients with IRC after 12 monthly IVIs have shown a higher risk for fibrosis and RPE atrophy compared with patients presenting refractory SRF [89]. By contrast, SRF is associated with stable VA, regardless of treatment frequency, and with better visual gain [50, 51, 90, 91]. Consequently, SRF is an ideal feature for identifying patients suitable for flexible or treat and extend regimens.

By contrast, SRF is associated with stable VA, regardless of treatment frequency, and with better visual gain, and consequently, is an ideal for flexible or treat and extend regimens [50, 51, 90, 91]. In conclusion, these subtypes tell us what outcomes we are hoping to achieve. We can personalize the treatment to some extent – treatment intervals can be maintained or extended where disease inactivity is achieved, i.e. IRF is improving or SRF is stable, or more agressive or in shortened intervals in patients with new and/or increased fluid. It is postulated that persistent IRF should never be tolerated whereas with persistent SRF we are less likely to treat until dry [92]. Advisably is also identifying patients with fluctuations in CSFT, who are convenient for closer monitoring and more aggressive therapy [28].

OCT-A may differentiate active CNV lesions from stable fibrous complexes which could be relevant for treatment decisions. Quantitative OCT-A parameters have shown as poor biomarkers in predicting anatomic and functional response although blood flow area and FD are slightly better than the others.

Recently, automated quantification algorithms have been proposed for the analysis of OCT images with CNV, namely multi-resolution graph-theoretic-based surface detection for PED segmentation and machine learning-based pixel classification for IRC and SRF segmentations [93]. Machine learning algorithms are particularly suitable for determining treatment effect after the loading phase [94]. Computational analysis of OCT images is expected to become even more widespread in the clinical treatment strategies. This will hopefully establish a set of standardized protocols that will allow personalized anti-VEGF treatments based on identifying important differences in retinal responses between patients.

Conflict of interest

The authors declare no conflict of interest.

Abbreviations

VEGF	vascular endothelial growth factor
AMD	age-related macular degeneration
nAMD	neovascular age-related macular degeneration
OCT	optical coherence tomography
CSFT	central subfoveal thickness
IRC	intraretinal cysts
SRF	subretinal fluid
PED	pigment epithelial detachment
sPED	serous
fvPED	fibrovascular
ELM	external limiting membrane
EZ	ellipsoid zone
RCT	randomized control trials
SD-OCT	spectral domain optical coherence tomography
IVT	intravitreal
IVI	intravitreal injection
CNV	choroidal neovascularization
RPE	retinal pigment epithelium
PRN	pro re nata (as needed)
TAE	treat-and-extend
ERM	epiretinal membrane
GA	geographic atrophy
RAP	retinal angiomatous proliferation
SHRM	subretinal hyperreflective material
NIR	near-infrared
OCT-A	optical coherence tomography angiography
SA	surface area
VD	vessel density
FD	fractal dimension
LAC	lacunarity index
FAZ	foveal avascular zone
FA	fluorescein angiography
IVGA	indocyanin green angiography
BM	Bruch membrane

Author details

Maja Vinković*, Andrijana Kopić and Tvrtka Benašić
Faculty of Medicine, Clinical Hospital Centre Osijek, Department of
Ophthalmology, Josip Juraj Strossmayer University of Osijek, Osijek, Croatia

*Address all correspondence to: majavinkovic77@gmail.com

IntechOpen

References

[1] Keane PA, Patel PJ, Liakopoulos S, Heussen FM, Sadda SR, Tufail A. Evaluation of age-related macular degeneration with optical coherence tomography. Surv Ophthalmol. 2012 Sep;57(5):389-414. doi: 10.1016/j. survophthal.2012.01.006.

[2] Mitchell P, Liew G, Gopinath B, Wong TY. Age-related macular degeneration. Lancet. 2018 Sep 29;392(10153):1147-1159. doi: 10.1016/ S0140-6736(18)31550-2.

[3] Wong WL, Su X, Li X, Cheung CM, Klein R, Cheng CY, Wong TY. Global prevalence of age-related macular degeneration and disease burden projection for 2020 and 2040: a systematic review and meta-analysis. Lancet Glob Health. 2014 Feb;2(2):e106-16. doi: 10.1016/ S2214-109X(13)70145-1.

[4] Holz FG, Schmitz-Valckenberg S, Fleckenstein M. Recent developments in the treatment of age-related macular degeneration. J Clin Invest. 2014 Apr;124(4):1430-8. doi: 10.1172/JCI71029.

[5] Wykoff CC, Clark WL, Nielsen JS, Brill JV, Greene LS, Heggen CL. Optimizing Anti-VEGF Treatment Outcomes for Patients with Neovascular Age-Related Macular Degeneration. J Manag Care Spec Pharm. 2018 Feb;24(2-a Suppl):S3-S15. doi: 10.18553/ jmcp.2018.24.2-a.s3.

[6] Bakri SJ, Thorne JE, Ho AC, Ehlers JP, Schoenberger SD, Yeh S, Kim SJ. Safety and Efficacy of Anti-Vascular Endothelial Growth Factor Therapies for Neovascular Age-Related Macular Degeneration: A Report by the American Academy of Ophthalmology. Ophthalmology. 2019 Jan;126(1):55-63. doi: 10.1016/j.ophtha.2018.07.028.

[7] Maguire MG, Martin DF, Ying GS, et al. Five-year outcomes with anti-vascular endothelial growth factor treatment of neovascular age-related macular degeneration: the Comparison of Age-Related Macular Degeneration Treatments Trials. Ophthalmology. 2016;123:1751e1761. doi: 10.1016/j. ophtha.2016.03.045

[8] Daniel E, Grunwald JE, Kim BJ, et al. Visual and morphologic outcomes in eyes with hard exudate in the comparison of agerelated macular degeneration treatments trials. Ophthalmol Retina. 2017;1:25-33. doi: 10.1016/j.oret.2016.09.001

[9] Ersoz MG, Karacorlu M, Arf S, et al. Retinal pigment epithelium tears: classification, pathogenesis, predictors, and management. Surv Ophthalmol. 2017;62:493-505. doi: 10.1016/j. survophthal.2017.03.004.

[10] Bhutto I, Lutty G. Understanding age-related macular degeneration (AMD): relationships between the photoreceptor/retinal pigment epithelium/Bruch's membrane/ choriocapillaris complex. Mol Aspects Med. 2012;33:295-317. doi: 10.1016/j. mam.2012.04.005

[11] Roh M, Selivanova A, Shin HJ, et al. Visual acuity and contrast sensitivity are two important factors affecting visionrelated quality of life in advanced age-related macular degeneration. PLoS One. 2018;13:e0196481. doi: 10.1371/ journal.pone.0196481.

[12] Mitchell J, Bradley C. Quality of life in age-related macular degeneration: a review of the literature. Health Qual Life Outcomes. 2006;4:97. doi: 10.1186/1477-7525-4-97.

[13] Mitchell P, Liew G, Gopinath B, Wong TY. Age-related macular degeneration. Lancet. 2018;392(10153): 1147-1159. doi: 10.1016/S0140-6736(18) 31550-2.

[14] Ferris FL, Wilkinson CP, Bird A, et al. Clinical classification of age-related macular degeneration. Ophthalmol. 2013;120(4):844-851. doi: 10.1016/j.ophtha.2012.10.036.

[15] Shibuya M. Vascular endothelial growth factor (VEGF) and its receptor (VEGFR) signaling in angiogenesis: a crucial target for anti- and pro-angiogenic therapies. Genes Cancer. 2011;2:1097-1105. doi: 10.1177/1947601911423031.

[16] Campochiaro PA, Aiello LP, Rosenfeld PJ. Anti-vascular endothelial growth factor agents in the treatment of retinal disease: from bench to bedside. Ophthalmology. 2016;123(10S):S78-S88. doi: 10.1016/j.ophtha.2016.04.056.

[17] Schmidt-Erfurth U, Chong V, Loewenstein A, et al. Guidelines for the management of neovascular age-related macular degeneration by the European Society of Retina Specialists (EURETINA). Br J Ophthalmol. 2014;98:1144-1167. doi: 10.1136/bjophthalmol-2014-305702.

[18] Gragoudas ES, Adamis AP, Cunningham Jr ET, et al. Pegaptanib for neovascular age-related macular degeneration. N Engl J Med. 2004;351:2805-2816. doi: 10.1056/NEJMoa042760.

[19] Brown DM, Kaiser PK, Michels M, et al. Ranibizumab versus verteporfin for neovascular age-related macular degeneration. N Engl J Med. 2006;355:1432-1444. doi: 10.1056/NEJMoa062655.

[20] Rosenfeld PJ, Brown DM, Heier JS, et al. Ranibizumab for neovascular age-related macular degeneration. N Engl J Med. 2006;355:1419-1431. doi: 10.1056/NEJMoa054481.

[21] Heier JS, Brown DM, Chong V, et al. Intravitreal aflibercept (VEGF trap-eye) in wet age-related macular degeneration. Ophthalmology. 2012;119:2537-2548. doi: 10.1016/j.ophtha.2012.09.006.

[22] Liu K, Song Y, Xu G, et al. Conbercept for treatment of neovascular age-related macular degeneration: results of the randomized phase 3 PHOENIX study. Am J Ophthalmol. 2019;197:156-167. doi: 10.1016/j.ajo.2018.08.026.

[23] de Oliveira Dias JR, de Andrade GC, Novais EA, et al. Fusion proteins for treatment of retinal diseases: aflibercept, ivaflibercept, and conbercept. Int J Retina Vitreous. 2016;2:3. doi: 10.1186/s40942-016-0026-y.

[24] Jaffe DH, Chan W, Bezlyak V, Skelly A. The economic and humanistic burden of patients in receipt of current available therapies for nAMD. J Comp Eff Res. 2018;7:1125-1132. doi: 10.2217/cer-2018-0058.

[25] Lanzetta P, Loewenstein A. Fundamental principles of an anti-VEGF treatment regimen: optimal application of intravitreal anti-vascular endothelial growth factor therapy of macular diseases. Graefes Arch Clin Exp Ophthalmol. 2017;255: 1259-1273. doi: 10.1007/s00417-017-3647-4.

[26] Ehlken C, Helms M, Bohringer D, et al. Association of treatment adherence with real-life VA outcomes in AMD, DME, and BRVO patients. Clin Ophthalmol. 2018;12:13-20. doi: 10.2147/OPTH.S151611.

[27] Wykoff CC, Croft DE, Brown DM, et al. Prospective trial of treat-and-extend versus monthly dosing for neovascular agerelated macular degeneration: TREX-AMD 1-year results. Ophthalmology. 2015;122:2514-2522. doi: 10.1016/j.ophtha.2015.08.009.

[28] Dugel PU, Koh A, Ogura Y, et al. HAWK and HARRIER: phase 3,

multicenter, randomized, double-masked trials of brolucizumab for neovascular age-related macular degeneration. Ophthalmology. 2020;127(1):72e84. doi: 10.1016/j.ophtha.2019.04.017.

[29] Leuschen JN, Schuman SG, Winter KP, McCall MN, Wong WT, Chew EY et al. Spectral-domain optical coherence tomography characteristics of intermediate age-related macular degeneration. Ophthalmology 2013; 120(1): 140-150. doi: 10.1016/j.ophtha.2012.07.004.

[30] Mcneil R. Considering the presence of retinal fluid when treating nAMD patients. Ophthalmology Times Europe. 2020. Vol. 16 No 6 6-9.

[31] Ma J, Desai R, Nesper P, Gill M, Fawzi A, Skondra D. Optical Coherence Tomographic Angiography Imaging in Age-Related Macular Degeneration. Ophthalmol Eye Dis. 2017;9: 1179172116686075. Published 2017 Mar 20. doi:10.1177/1179172116686075

[32] Nagiel A, Sadda SR, Sarraf D. A promising future for optical coherence tomography angiography. JAMA Ophthalmol. 2015;133:629-630. doi: 10.1001/jamaophthalmol.2015.0668.

[33] Fang PP, Lindner M, Steinberg JS, et al. Clinical applications of OCT angiography. Ophthalmologe. 2016;113:14-22.

[34] Cheung CMG, Grewal DS, Teo KYC, Gan A, Mohla A, Chakravarthy U, Wong TY, Jaffe GJ. The Evolution of Fibrosis and Atrophy and Their Relationship with Visual Outcomes in Asian Persons with Neovascular Age-Related Macular Degeneration. Ophthalmol Retina. 2019 Dec;3(12):1045-1055. doi: 10.1016/j.oret.2019.06.002.

[35] Willoughby AS, Ying GS, Toth CA, Maguire MG, Burns RE, Grunwald JE,

Daniel E, Jaffe GJ; Comparison of Age-Related Macular Degeneration Treatments Trials Research Group. Subretinal Hyperreflective Material in the Comparison of Age-Related Macular Degeneration Treatments Trials. Ophthalmology. 2015 Sep;122(9):1846-53.e5. doi: 10.1016/j.ophtha.2015.05.042.

[36] Daniel E, Shaffer J, Ying GS, Grunwald JE, Martin DF, Jaffe GJ, Maguire MG; Comparison of Age-Related Macular Degeneration Treatments Trials (CATT) Research Group. Outcomes in Eyes with Retinal Angiomatous Proliferation in the Comparison of Age-Related Macular Degeneration Treatments Trials (CATT). Ophthalmology. 2016 Mar;123(3):609-16. doi: 10.1016/j.ophtha.2015.10.034

[37] Daniel E, Toth CA, Grunwald JE, Jaffe GJ, Martin DF, Fine SL, Huang J, Ying GS, Hagstrom SA, Winter K, Maguire MG; Comparison of Age-related Macular Degeneration Treatments Trials Research Group. Risk of scar in the comparison of age-related macular degeneration treatments trials. Ophthalmology. 2014 Mar;121(3):656-66. doi: 10.1016/j.ophtha.2013.10.019.

[38] Freund KB, Ho IV, Barbazetto IA et al. Type 3 neovascularization: the expanded spectrum of retinal angiomatous proliferation. Retina. 2008 Feb;28(2):201-11. doi: 10.1097/IAE.0b013e3181669504.

[39] Yanuzzi LA, Negrao S, Iida T, et al. Retinal angiomatous proliferation in age-related macular degeneration. Retina 2012;32(Suppl 1):416-34. doi: 10.1097/iae.0b013e31823f9b3b

[40] Browning AC, O'Brien JM, Vieira RV, Gupta R, Nenova K. Intravitreal Aflibercept for Retinal Angiomatous Proliferation: Results of a Prospective Case Series at 96 Weeks. Ophthalmologica. 2019;242(4):239-246. doi: 10.1159/000500203

[41] Schmidt-Erfurth U, Waldstein SM. A paradigm shift in imaging biomarkers in neovascular age-related macular degeneration. Prog Retin Eye Res. 2016;50:1-24. doi: 10.1016/j.preteyeres.2015.07.007.

[42] Amoaku WM, Chakravarthy U, Gale R, Gavin M, Ghanchi F, Gibson J, Harding S, Johnston RL, Kelly SP, Lotery A, Mahmood S, Menon G, Sivaprasad S, Talks J, Tufail A, Yang Y. Defining response to anti-VEGF therapies in neovascular AMD. Eye (Lond). 2015 Jun;29(6):721-31. doi: 10.1038/eye.2015.48.

[43] Grunwald JE, Pistilli M, Daniel E, Ying GS, Pan W, Jaffe GJ, Toth CA, Hagstrom SA, Maguire MG, Martin DF; Comparison of Age-Related Macular Degeneration Treatments Trials Research Group. Incidence and Growth of Geographic Atrophy during 5 Years of Comparison of Age-Related Macular Degeneration Treatments Trials. Ophthalmology. 2017 Jan;124(1):97-104. doi: 10.1016/j.ophtha.2016.09.012.

[44] Lai TT, Hsieh YT, Yang CM, Ho TC, Yang CH. Biomarkers of optical coherence tomography in evaluating the treatment outcomes of neovascular age-related macular degeneration: a real-world study. Sci Rep. 2019 Jan 24;9(1):529. doi: 10.1038/s41598-018-36704-6.

[45] Schmidt-Erfurth U, Eldem B, Guymer R, Korobelnik JF, Schlingemann RO, Axer-Siegel R, Wiedemann P, Simader C, Gekkieva M, Weichselberger A; EXCITE Study Group. Efficacy and safety of monthly versus quarterly ranibizumab treatment in neovascular age-related macular degeneration: the EXCITE study. Ophthalmology. 2011 May;118(5):831-9. doi: 10.1016/j.ophtha.2010.09.004.

[46] Waldstein, S. M. et al. Morphology and Visual Acuity in Aflibercept and Ranibizumab Therapy for Neovascular

Age-Related Macular Degeneration in the VIEW Trials. Ophthalmology 123, 1521-1529 (2016) doi: 10.1016/j.ophtha.2016.03.037

[47] Simader C, Ritter M, Bolz M, Deák GG, Mayr-Sponer U, Golbaz I, Kundi M, Schmidt-Erfurth UM. Morphologic parameters relevant for visual outcome during anti-angiogenic therapy of neovascular age-related macular degeneration. Ophthalmology. 2014 Jun;121(6):1237-45. doi: 10.1016/j.ophtha.2013.12.029.

[48] Tan CS, Lim LW, Ngo WK, et al. Predictors of persistent disease activity following anti-VEGF loading dose for nAMD patients in Singapore: the DIALS study. BMC Ophthalmol. 2020;20(1):324. Published 2020 Aug 6. doi:10.1186/s12886-020-01582-y

[49] Clemens CR, Alten F, Termühlen J, et al. Prospective PED-study of intravitreal aflibercept for refractory vascularized pigment epithelium detachment due to age-related macular degeneration: morphologic characteristics of non-responders in optical coherence tomography. Graefes Arch Clin Exp Ophthalmol. 2020;258(7):1411-1417. doi:10.1007/s00417-020-04675-y

[50] Arnold JJ, Markey CM, Kurstjens NP, Guymer RH. The role of sub-retinal fluid in determining treatment outcomes in patients with neovascular age-related macular degeneration--a phase IV randomised clinical trial with ranibizumab: the FLUID study. BMC Ophthalmol. 2016 Mar 24;16:31. doi: 10.1186/s12886-016-0207-3.

[51] Veritti D, Sarao V, Missiroli F, Ricci F, Lanzetta P. TWELVE-MONTH OUTCOMES OF INTRAVITREAL AFLIBERCEPT FOR NEOVASCULAR AGE-RELATED MACULAR DEGENERATION: Fixed Versus As-needed Dosing. Retina. 2019

Nov;39(11):2077-2083. doi: 10.1097/
IAE.0000000000002299

[52] Pron G. Optical Coherence
Tomography Monitoring Strategies for
A-VEGF-Treated Age-Related Macular
Degeneration: An Evidence-Based
Analysis. Ont Health Technol Assess Ser.
2014;14(10):1-64. Published 2014 Aug 1.

[53] Inan S, Polat O, Karadas M,
Inan UU. The association of exudation
pattern with anatomical and functional
outcomes in patients with Neovascular
Age-Related Macular Degeneration.
Rom J Ophthalmol. 2019;63(3):238-244.

[54] Mantel I, Niderprim SA,
Gianniou C, Deli A, Ambresin A.
Reducing the clinical burden of
ranibizumab treatment for neovascular
age-related macular degeneration using
an individually planned regimen. Br J
Ophthalmol. 2014;98(9):1192-1196.
doi:10.1136/bjophthalmol-2013-304556

[55] Ashraf, M., Souka, A. & Adelman,
R. A. Age-related macular degeneration:
using morphological predictors to
modify current treatment protocols.
Acta Ophthalmol. 96, 120-133 (2018).
doi: 10.1111/aos.13565.

[56] Cheong KX, Teo KYC,
Cheung CMG. Influence of pigment
epithelial detachment on visual acuity in
neovascular age-related macular
degeneration. Surv Ophthalmol. 2021
Jan-Feb;66(1):68-97. doi: 10.1016/j.
survophthal.2020.05.003.

[57] Balaskas K, Karampelas M,
Horani M, et al. Quantitative analysis of
pigment epithelial detachment response
to different anti-vascular endothelial
growth factor agents in wet age-related
macular degeneration. Retina. 2017
Jul;37(7):1297-304. doi: 10.1097/
IAE.0000000000001342.

[58] Tyagi, P., Juma, Z., Hor, Y.K. et al.
Clinical response of pigment epithelial
detachment associated with neovascular

age-related macular degeneration in
switching treatment from Ranibizumab
to Aflibercept. BMC Ophthalmol 18, 148
(2018). doi: 10.1186/s12886-018-0824-0.

[59] Karampelas M, Malamos P, Petrou P,
Georgalas I, Papaconstantinou D,
Brouzas D. Retinal Pigment Epithelial
Detachment in Age-Related Macular
Degeneration. Ophthalmol Ther.
2020;9(4):739-756. doi:10.1007/
s40123-020-00291-5

[60] Nagai N, Suzuki M, Uchida A, et al.
Non-responsiveness to intravitreal
aflibercept treatment in neovascular
age-related macular degeneration:
implications of serous pigment
epithelial detachment. Sci Rep.
2016;6:29619. Published 2016 Jul 11.
doi:10.1038/srep29619

[61] Malihi M, Jia Y, Gao SS, et al.
Optical coherence tomographic
angiography of choroidal
neovascularization ill-defined with
fluorescein angiography. Br J
Ophthalmol. 2017;101(1):45-50.
doi:10.1136/bjophthalmol-2016-309094

[62] Khanani AM, Eichenbaum D,
Schlottmann PG, Tuomi L, Sarraf D.
OPTIMAL MANAGEMENT OF
PIGMENT EPITHELIAL
DETACHMENTS IN EYES WITH
NEOVASCULAR AGE-RELATED
MACULAR DEGENERATION. Retina.
2018;38(11):2103-2117. doi:10.1097/
IAE.0000000000002195

[63] Laishram M, Srikanth K,
Rajalakshmi AR, Nagarajan S,
Ezhumalai G. Microperimetry - A New
Tool for Assessing Retinal Sensitivity in
Macular Diseases. J Clin Diagn Res.
2017;11(7):NC08-NC11. doi:10.7860/
JCDR/2017/25799.10213

[64] Suzuki M, Nagai N, Izumi-Nagai K,
Shinoda H, Koto T, Uchida A,
Mochimaru H, Yuki K, Sasaki M,
Tsubota K, Ozawa Y. Predictive factors
for non-response to intravitreal

ranibizumab treatment in age-related macular degeneration. Br J Ophthalmol. 2014 Sep;98(9):1186-91. doi: 10.1136/bjophthalmol-2013-304670

[65] Hoerster, R., Muether, P. S., Sitnilska, V., Kirchhof, B. & Fauser, S. Fibrovascular pigment epithelial detachment is a risk factor for long-term visual decay in neovascular age-related macular degeneretion. Retina 34, 1767-1773 (2014). doi: 10.1097/IAE.0000000000000188.

[66] Au A, Hou K, Dávila JP, Gunnemann F, Fragiotta S, Arya M, Sacconi R, Pauleikhoff D, Querques G, Waheed N, Freund KB, Sadda S, Sarraf D. Volumetric Analysis of Vascularized Serous Pigment Epithelial Detachment Progression in Neovascular Age-Related Macular Degeneration Using Optical Coherence Tomography Angiography. Invest Ophthalmol Vis Sci. 2019 Aug 1;60(10):3310-3319. doi: 10.1167/iovs.18-26478

[67] Juma Z, Hor YK, Scott NW, Ionean A, Santiago C. Clinical response of pigment epithelial detachment associated with neovascular age-related macular degeneration in switching treatment from Ranibizumab to Aflibercept. BMC Ophthalmol. 2018;18(1):148. Published 2018 Jun 22. doi:10.1186/s12886-018-0824-0

[68] Punjabi OS, Huang J, Rodriguez L, Lyon AT, Jampol LM, Mirza RG. Imaging characteristics of neovascular pigment epithelial detachments and their response to anti-vascular endothelial growth factor therapy. Br J Ophthalmol. 2013 Aug;97(8):1024-31. doi: 10.1136/bjophthalmol-2013-303155

[69] Tarakcioglu HN, Ozkaya A, Kemer B, Taskapili M. Multimodal imaging based biomarkers predictive of early and late response to anti-VEGFs during the first year of treatment for neovascular age-related macular degeneration. J Fr Ophtalmol. 2019 Jan;42(1):22-31. doi: 10.1016/j.jfo.2018.06.005.

[70] de Massougnes S, Dirani A, Mantel I. GOOD VISUAL OUTCOME AT 1 YEAR IN NEOVASCULAR AGE-RELATED MACULAR DEGENERATION WITH PIGMENT EPITHELIUM DETACHMENT: Factors Influencing the Treatment Response. Retina. 2018 Apr;38(4):717-724. doi: 10.1097/IAE.0000000000001613.

[71] Clemens CR, Krohne TU, Charbel Issa P, Helb HM, Kosanetzky N, Lommatzsch A, Holz FG, Eter N. High-resolution optical coherence tomography of subpigment epithelial structures in patients with pigment epithelium detachment secondary to age-related macular degeneration. Br J Ophthalmol. 2012 Aug;96(8):1088-91. doi: 10.1136/bjophthalmol-2011-301415.

[72] Leitritz M, Gelisken F, Inhoffen W, Voelker M, Ziemssen F. Can the risk of retinal pigment epithelium tears after bevacizumab treatment be predicted? An optical coherence tomography study. Eye (Lond). 2008 Dec;22(12):1504-7. doi: 10.1038/eye.2008.145.

[73] Faatz H, Farecki ML, Rothaus K, Gutfleisch M, Pauleikhoff D, Lommatzsch A. Changes in the OCT angiographic appearance of type 1 and type 2 CNV in exudative AMD during anti-VEGF treatment. BMJ Open Ophthalmol. 2019 Dec 10;4(1):e000369. doi: 10.1136/bmjophth-2019-000369.

[74] Clemens CR, Bastian N, Alten F, Milojcic C, Heiduschka P, Eter N. Prediction of retinal pigment epithelial tear in serous vascularized pigment epithelium detachment. Acta Ophthalmol. 2014 Feb;92(1):e50-6. doi: 10.1111/aos.12234.

[75] Coscas GJ, Lupidi M, Coscas F, Cagini C, Souied EH. OPTICAL COHERENCE TOMOGRAPHY ANGIOGRAPHY VERSUS

TRADITIONAL MULTIMODAL IMAGING IN ASSESSING THE ACTIVITY OF EXUDATIVE AGE-RELATED MACULAR DEGENERATION: A New Diagnostic Challenge. Retina. 2015 Nov;35(11):2219-28. doi: 10.1097/IAE.0000000000000766.

[76] Nikolopoulou E, Lorusso M, Micelli Ferrari L, Cicinelli MV, Bandello F, Querques G, Micelli Ferrari T. Optical Coherence Tomography Angiography versus Dye Angiography in Age-Related Macular Degeneration: Sensitivity and Specificity Analysis. Biomed Res Int. 2018 Mar 7;2018:6724818. doi: 10.1155/2018/6724818.

[77] Huang D, Jia Y, Rispoli M, Tan O, Lumbroso B. OPTICAL COHERENCE TOMOGRAPHY ANGIOGRAPHY OF TIME COURSE OF CHOROIDAL NEOVASCULARIZATION IN RESPONSE TO ANTI-ANGIOGENIC TREATMENT. Retina. 2015 Nov;35(11):2260-4. doi: 10.1097/IAE.0000000000000846.

[78] Perrott-Reynolds R, Cann R, Cronbach N, Neo YN, Ho V, McNally O, Madi HA, Cochran C, Chakravarthy U. The diagnostic accuracy of OCT angiography in naive and treated neovascular age-related macular degeneration: a review. Eye (Lond). 2019 Feb;33(2):274-282. doi: 10.1038/s41433-018-0229-6.

[79] Coscas F, Lupidi M, Boulet JF, et al. Optical coherence tomography angiography in exudative age-related macular degeneration: a predictive model for treatment decisions. Br J Ophthalmol. 2019;103: 1342-1346. doi:10.1136/bjophthalmol-2018-313065

[80] Stattin M, Forster J, Daniel A, Graf A, Krepler K, Ansari-Shahrezaei S. Relationship between Neovascular Density in Swept Source-Optical Coherence Tomography Angiography and Signs of Activity in Exudative Age-Related Macular Degeneration. J Ophthalmol. 2019;2019:4806061. Published 2019 Jul 9. doi:10.1155/2019/4806061

[81] McClintic SM, Gao S, Wang J, Hagag A, Lauer AK, Flaxel CJ, Bhavsar K, Hwang TS, Huang D, Jia Y, Bailey ST. Quantitative Evaluation of Choroidal Neovascularization under Pro Re Nata Anti-Vascular Endothelial Growth Factor Therapy with OCT Angiography. Ophthalmol Retina. 2018 Sep;2(9):931-941. doi: 10.1016/j.oret.2018.01.014.

[82] Spaide RF, Fujimoto JG, Waheed NK. IMAGE ARTIFACTS IN OPTICAL COHERENCE TOMOGRAPHY ANGIOGRAPHY. Retina. 2015 Nov; 35(11):2163-80. doi: 10.1097/IAE.0000000000000765.

[83] Cabral D, Coscas F, Pereira T, Français C, Geraldes C, Laiginhas R, Rodrigues C, Kashi AK, Nogueira V, Falcão M, Papoila AL, Lupidi M, 19.Coscas G, Cohen SY, Souied E. Quantitative Optical Coherence Tomography Angiography Biomarkers in a Treat-and-Extend Dosing Regimen in Neovascular Age-Related Macular Degeneration. Transl Vis Sci Technol. 2020 Feb 14;9(3):18. doi: 10.1167/tvst.9.3.18.

[84] Al-Sheikh M, Iafe NA, Phasukkijwatana N, Sadda SR, Sarraf D. Biomarkers of neovascular activity in age-related macular degeneration using OCT angiography. Retina. 2018; 38: 220-230. doi:10.1097/IAE.0000000000001628

[85] Roberts PK, Nesper PL, Gill MK, Fawzi AA. SEMIAUTOMATED QUANTITATIVE APPROACH TO CHARACTERIZE TREATMENT RESPONSE IN NEOVASCULAR AGE-RELATED MACULAR DEGENERATION: A Real-World Study. Retina. 2017 Aug; 37(8):1492-1498. doi: 10.1097/IAE.0000000000001400

[86] Corvi F, Pellegrini M, Erba S, Cozzi M, Staurenghi G, Giani A. Reproducibility of Vessel Density, Fractal Dimension, and Foveal Avascular Zone Using 7 Different Optical Coherence Tomography Angiography Devices. Am J Ophthalmol. 2018 Feb;186:25-31. doi: 10.1016/j.ajo.2017.11.011.

[87] Nguyen V, Daien V, Guymer R, Young S, Hunyor A, Fraser-Bell S, Hunt A, Gillies MC, Barthelmes D; Fight Retinal Blindness! Study Group. Projection of Long-Term Visual Acuity Outcomes Based on Initial Treatment Response in Neovascular Age-Related Macular Degeneration. Ophthalmology. 2019 Jan;126(1):64-74. doi: 10.1016/j. ophtha.2018.08.023. Epub 2018 Aug 24. PMID: 30149035.

[88] de Moura J, L Vidal P, Novo J, Rouco J, G Penedo M, Ortega M. Intraretinal Fluid Pattern Characterization in Optical Coherence Tomography Images. Sensors (Basel). 2020 Apr 3;20(7):2004. doi: 10.3390/s20072004.

[89] Mitchell P, Korobelnik JF, Lanzetta P, Holz FG, Prünte C, Schmidt-Erfurth U, Tano Y, Wolf S. Ranibizumab (Lucentis) in neovascular age-related macular degeneration: evidence from clinical trials. Br J Ophthalmol. 2010 Jan;94(1):2-13. doi: 10.1136/bjo.2009.159160.

[90] Penha FM, Gregori G, Garcia Filho CA, Yehoshua Z, Feuer WJ, Rosenfeld PJ. Quantitative changes in retinal pigment epithelial detachments as a predictor for retreatment with anti-VEGF therapy. Retina. 2013 Mar;33(3):459-66. doi: 10.1097/IAE.0b013e31827d2657

[91] Akagi-Kurashige Y, Tsujikawa A, Oishi A, Ooto S, Yamashiro K, Tamura H, Nakata I, Ueda-Arakawa N, Yoshimura N. Relationship between retinal morphological findings and visual function in age-related macular degeneration. Graefes Arch Clin Exp Ophthalmol. 2012 Aug;250(8):1129-36. doi: 10.1007/s00417-012-1928-5.

[92] Sharma S, Toth CA, Daniel E, Grunwald JE, Maguire MG, Ying GS, et al. Macular morphology and visual acuity in the second year of the comparison of age-related macular degeneration treatments trials. Ophthalmology. 2016;123:865-75. doi: 10.1016/j.ophtha.2015.12.002.

[93] Xiayu Xu, Kyungmoo Lee, Li Zhang, Sonka M, Abramoff MD. Stratified Sampling Voxel Classification for Segmentation of Intraretinal and Subretinal Fluid in Longitudinal Clinical OCT Data. IEEE Trans Med Imaging. 2015 Jul;34(7):1616-1623. doi: 10.1109/TMI.2015.2408632

[94] Bogunovic H, Abramoff M, Zhang L, Sonka M. Prediction of Treatment Response from Retinal OCT in Patients with Exudative Age-Related Macular Degeneration. International Workshop on Ophthalmic Medical Image Analysis of MICCAI: Boston,MA, USA, 2014.

Chapter 5

New Drugs in the Pipeline for the Management of AMD

Ana Marta and Bernardete Pessoa

Abstract

Anti-vascular endothelial growth factor (anti-VEGF) therapies have revolutionized the care of patients with retinal diseases. In the 1990s, it was observed that anti-VEGF antibodies reduced tumor angiogenesis, and consequently, these antibodies started to be used off-label in the exudative form of age-related macular degeneration (AMD). In the 2000s, research was directed towards the development of anti-VEGF therapies for retinal disease management. Several anti-VEGF therapies were approved: pegaptanib, an RNA aptamer, in 2004; ranibizumab, an anti-VEGF F_{ab}, in 2008; aflibercept, a humanized IgG F_c, in 2011; and brolucizumab, an scFv, in 2019. Currently, new therapeutic options are emerging, and approval is expected soon. These new therapies aim to increase treatment durability and thus reduce treatment burden and improve real-world outcomes. In this chapter, the mechanisms of action and the preliminary trial results of these potential new therapies will be described.

Keywords: AMD, drug therapy, intravitreal injections, clinical trials, pipeline

1. Introduction

Global prevalence estimates suggest that approximately 196 million people lived with age-related macular degeneration (AMD) in 2020. Of these, 10.4 million people were living with moderate to severe vision impairment. In 2030, AMD is estimated to affect 243 million people due to aging [1]. The pathogenesis of AMD results from complex multifactorial interactions, including metabolic, genetic, and environmental [2]. AMD has been classified into two major subtypes: non-exudative or dry AMD and exudative or wet AMD. Although dry AMD represents 90% of patients, exudative AMD causes more severe loss of vision, being the target of most investigations [3]. These patients require very regular clinic visits, and the chronicity of anti-vascular endothelial growth factor (anti-VEGF) therapy can substantially impact the quality of life of the patient and the caregivers [4, 5]. This decrease can compromise anti-VEGF therapy compliance and explain the undertreatment of patients observed in real-world studies and the waiver of patients involved in clinical trials [6, 7]. New trials are focusing on improving the therapeutic options, particularly on the decrease of the associated burden. This chapter describes the current research on therapeutical approaches to treat the dry and exudative forms of AMD. **Figure 1** summarizes the drugs and stages of development.

The information was gathered from a medical literature review and ongoing clinical trials and their results in the area of AMD treatment using PubMed database (https://www.ncbi.nlm.nih.gov/pubmed). The words or medical head subjects

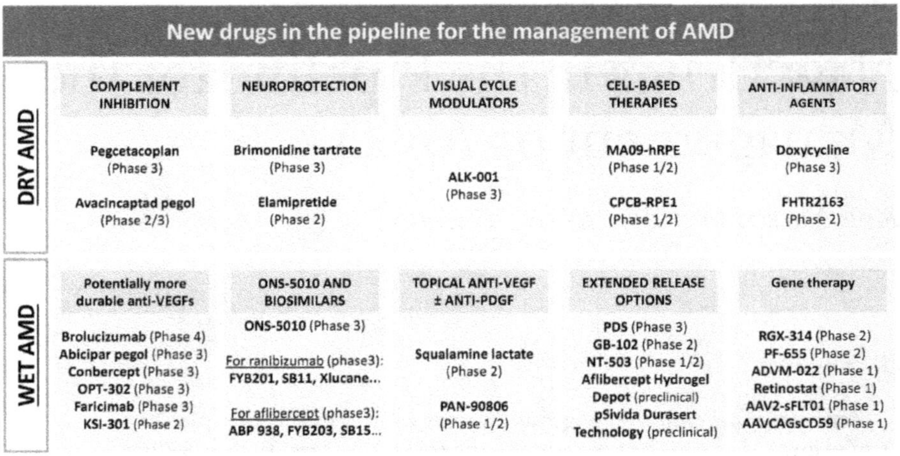

New drugs in the pipeline for the management of AMD

	COMPLEMENT INHIBITION	NEUROPROTECTION	VISUAL CYCLE MODULATORS	CELL-BASED THERAPIES	ANTI-INFLAMMATORY AGENTS
DRY AMD	Pegcetacoplan (Phase 3) Avacincaptad pegol (Phase 2/3)	Brimonidine tartrate (Phase 3) Elamipretide (Phase 2)	ALK-001 (Phase 3)	MA09-hRPE (Phase 1/2) CPCB-RPE1 (Phase 1/2)	Doxycycline (Phase 3) FHTR2163 (Phase 2)

	Potentially more durable anti-VEGFs	ONS-5010 AND BIOSIMILARS	TOPICAL ANTI-VEGF ± ANTI-PDGF	EXTENDED RELEASE OPTIONS	Gene therapy
WET AMD	Brolucizumab (Phase 4) Abicipar pegol (Phase 3) Conbercept (Phase 3) OPT-302 (Phase 3) Faricimab (Phase 3) KSI-301 (Phase 2)	ONS-5010 (Phase 3) For ranibizumab (phase3): FYB201, SB11, Xlucane... For aflibercept (phase3): ABP 938, FYB203, SB15...	Squalamine lactate (Phase 2) PAN-90806 (Phase 1/2)	PDS (Phase 3) GB-102 (Phase 2) NT-503 (Phase 1/2) Aflibercept Hydrogel Depot (preclinical) pSivida Durasert Technology (preclinical)	RGX-314 (Phase 2) PF-655 (Phase 2) ADVM-022 (Phase 1) Retinostat (Phase 1) AAV2-sFLT01 (Phase 1) AAVCAGsCD59 (Phase 1)

Figure 1.
Summary of new drugs in the pipeline for the management of age-related macular degeneration (AMD).

used were: AMD and clinical trials. All relevant articles were imported into Zotero (Version 5.0, Center for History and New Media at Universidade George Mason, USA), and duplicate articles were deleted. We selected the promising therapies according to action mechanisms and excluded all therapies that had failed in clinical trials. Comments, editorials, and articles not written in English were not analyzed.

2. For dry AMD

2.1 Complement inhibition

Although lampalizumab (anti-factor D Fab) and eculizumab (inhibitor of the activation of terminal complement) failed to slow geographic atrophy progression, the complement system has been implicated in the pathogenesis of geographic atrophy, and so, research on how to inhibit the complement system did not stop [8, 9].

Pegcetacoplan (APL-2; Apellis Pharmaceuticals, Waltham, Massachusetts, USA) is a synthetic molecule that selectively inhibits C3, effectively downregulating all three complement pathways. Phase 2 of the FILLY clinical trial compared patients receiving intravitreal injection (monthly and bi-monthly) with a control group. The results showed a 29% reduction in the rate of geographic atrophy and a better outcome in the monthly injection group. Moreover, it was observed that the risk of neovascular AMD was higher (18%) in the group subjected to monthly injections when comparing with the group subjected to bi-monthly injections (8%) and with the control group (1%) [10]. A phase 3 trial is currently in the recruitment phase (NCT03525600) [11].

Avacincaptad pegol (Zimura; Iveric Bio, New York, New York, USA) is a C5 inhibitor. Phase 2/3 GATHER1 clinical trial showed a significant reduction of geographic atrophy growth over 12 months, probably due to C3 activity preservation. A second confirmatory trial (GATHER2) is underway [12].

2.2 Neuroprotection

Retinal neuroprotection strategies have been studied for dry AMD, including apoptosis and necrosis prevention, and oxidative injury reduction [13].

Elamipretide (Stealth Biotherapeutics) is a mitochondria-targeted drug thought to reduce mitochondrial dysfunction. Phase 1 of the ReCLAIM clinical trial showed that elamipretide was safe, well-tolerated and that this drug may improve vision in patients with intermediate AMD, manifested as high-risk drusen [14]. Phase 2 ReCLAIM-2 clinical trial is underway [15].

Brimonidine tartrate (Allergan) is best known in glaucoma as the intraocular pressure (IOP) lowering agent. Phase 2A of the BEACON clinical trial assessed the intravitreally delivery of brimonidine through a delayed delivery system. Results showed a lower rate of geographic atrophy progression, although not statistically significant [16]. Phase 2B of the BEACON clinical trial demonstrated a reduction in geographic atrophy progression using higher doses of brimonidine [17]. Phase 3 of IMAGINE and ENVISION clinical trials are being designed [16].

2.3 Visual cycle modulators

One of the earliest changes in the retina that precede AMD symptoms is the formation of toxic vitamin A dimers.

ALK-001 (Alkeus Pharmaceuticals) is a chemically modified form of vitamin A that replaces the vitamin A in the body to prevent toxic vitamin A dimers. Studies demonstrated functional preservation of visual function in animal models [18]. Phase 3 of the SAGA clinical trial will measure the extent to which treatment with the oral capsule of ALK-001 slows geographic atrophy progression [19].

2.4 Cell-based therapies

Cell therapy is an alternative strategy when the naturally existing cells are already too damaged to be preserved using neuroprotective agents. Human pluripotent stem cells (hPSCs) comprise human embryonic stem cells (hESCs) and human-induced pluripotent stem cells (hiPSCs). There are two subtypes of cell-based treatments: stem cell therapies that involve delivering new retinal pigment epithelial (RPE) cells to the subretinal space, and non-stem cell therapies based on cell implantation, which generates protective factors [20].

MA09-hRPE (Astellas Pharma) is hESC-derived Retinal Pigment Epithelium (hESC-RPE). The phases 1/2 clinical trial results confirmed that hESC-derived cells could serve as a potentially safe new source for regenerative medicine [21–23].

CPCB-RPE1 (The California Project to Cure Blindness-Retinal Pigment Epithelium1) is a polarized monolayer of hESC-RPE ultrathin, synthetic parylene substrate designed to mimic Bruch's membrane. This therapy involves a subretinal implant. It was demonstrated the feasibility and safety of CPCB-RPE1 subretinal implantation in a comparable animal model [24]. Phase 1/2A of the clinical trial suggests that CPCB-RPE1 may improve visual function [25, 26].

2.5 Anti-inflammatory agents

Inflammation has been implicated in AMD pathogenesis and progression, even though it is no classical inflammatory disease like uveitis [27].

Doxycycline (Oracea; Galderma Laboratories, Fort Worth, Texas, USA) is an antibiotic that belongs to the tetracycline class of antibiotics and plays a role in immunomodulation, cell proliferation, angiogenesis, and the regulation of inflammation. Phase 3 of the TOGA clinical trial includes patients with geographic atrophy randomized in groups treated with Oracea® or placebo. The results are pending [28].

FHTR2163 (Genentech/Roche) is a new antibody delivered by intravitreal injection that inhibits the HTRA1 gene associated with geographic atrophy. Phase 2 of the GALLEGO clinical trial will evaluate the safety, tolerability, and efficacy of intravitreal injections of RG6147, administered every four or every eight weeks for a total of approximately 76 weeks, in participants with geographic atrophy secondary to AMD (when compared with the sham control) [29].

3. For wet AMD

3.1 Potentially more durable anti-VEGF agents

Potentially more durable anti-VEGF agents may reduce the burden of intravitreal injections, help stabilize the disease and improve compliance with treatment.

Brolucizumab (Beovu; Novartis, Basel, Switzerland) is the most recent intravitreal anti-VEGF agent to receive FDA approval. It is a humanized single-chain antibody fragment with a molecular weight of 26 kDa. Phase 3 of the HAWK and HARRIER clinical trials showed that brolucizumab was non-inferior to aflibercept regarding visual function as at week 48, more than 50% of the eyes treated with 6 mg of brolucizumab were maintained on q12w dosing intervals. Moreover, anatomic outcomes favored brolucizumab over aflibercept, and the overall safety results were similar between the two drugs [30].

Abicipar pegol (Allergan) is a novel class of molecules referred to as designed ankyrin repeat proteins (DARPin) that bind VEGF-A. DARPin is smaller and has a high affinity to VEGF, leading to greater stability and a longer-acting effect. The results of phase 3 of the SEQUOIA and CEDAR clinical trials showed that the eight and 12-week abicipar regimens were non-inferior to the ranibizumab's monthly regimen, but patients had a much higher risk of developing intraocular inflammation (15% and 15.4% vs. 0%) [31–33]. The company modified the manufacturing process after finding impurities in the formulation, and subsequently, the MAPLE study showed a decrease in the incidence of intraocular inflammation to 8.9% [34]. A license for abicipar pegol was already submitted to the *Food and Drug Administration* and the European Medicines Agency.

Conbercept (Chengdu Kanghong Biotech Co., Ltd.) is an antibody that targets VEGF-A, VEGFB, VEGF-C, and placental growth factors. It was approved to treat exudative AMD in China in 2013. Phase 2 of the AURORA and phase 3 of the PHOENIX clinical trials showed the safety and efficacy of conbercept with three initial monthly treatments followed by quarterly treatments compared with the sham group [35, 36]. Phase 3 of the PANDA-1 and PANDA-2 global clinical trials compare maintenance doses of conbercept every 8 or 12 weeks with doses of aflibercept every eight weeks; results are expected in 2022 [37, 38].

OPT-302 (Opthea Limited) is a soluble form of the human VEGF receptor-3 (VEGFR-3), expressed as an Fc-fusion protein molecule design to inhibit VEGF-C and VEGF-D. Results from phases 1 and 2 of the ShORe and COAST clinical trials showed that this molecule was safer and had better visual outcomes than ranibizumab alone [39, 40]. Phase 3 of the ShORe and COAST clinical trials will be double-masked and sham-controlled. Treatment-naïve patients will be enrolled to assess the efficacy and safety of 2.0 mg OPT-302 combined with anti-VEGF-A therapy by comparison with anti-VEGF-A monotherapy (standard of care). Opthea expects to initiate patient recruitment in the first half of 2021 [41].

Faricimab (Roche, Genentech) is a novel bispecific antibody that targets both angiopoietin-2 (Ang-2) and VEGF-A. Phase 2 of the STAIRWAY clinical trial suggests that faricimab can be an effective maintenance therapy for exudative AMD with a dosing interval of 16 weeks [42, 43]. Phase 3 of the TANAYA and LUCERNE clinical trials will compare faricimab given every 16 weeks with aflibercept given every eight weeks [44, 45]. FDA requests for faricimab are expected to occur in 2021 for diabetic macular edema and in 2022 for exudative AMD.

KSI-301 (Kodiak Sciences) is a novel intravitreal, anti-VEGF antibody biopolymer conjugate designed to block all VEGF-A isoforms. Phase 1 of the DAZZLE clinical trial showed excellent safety, strong efficacy, and considerable durability in most patients for three or more months [46]. Phase 2 of the DAZZLE clinical trial is a prospective, randomized controlled clinical trial designed to evaluate the safety and efficacy of KSI-301 [47].

3.2 ONS-5010 and biosimilars

ONS-5010 (Outlook Therapeutics, Inc) is an ophthalmic formulation of bevacizumab. Phase 3 clinical trials compare monthly doses of ONS-5010 with a ranibizumab regimen of 3 monthly doses followed by quarterly doses [48]. FDA approval is expected in 2021 or 2022, and 12 years of exclusivity, protecting against bevacizumab biosimilars, are expected.

FYB201 (Formycon and Bioeq), SB11 (Samsung Bioepis), and Xlucane (Xbrane Biopharma) are biosimilars for ranibizumab under development that are expected to reach the market in less than one year when the patent for ranibizumab expires [49–51].

Aflibercept biosimilars are in phase 3 of clinical trials and are expected to reach the market between two and three years when the patent for aflibercept expires.

3.3 Topical anti-VEGF ± anti-PDGF

Although regorafenib, pazopanib, and LHA510 failed, other therapies showed promising results [52–54]. These formulations have the great advantage of being less invasive, but they can decrease the possibility of monitoring treatment compliance, as it happens with glaucoma patients medicated with lowering ocular hypertension drops.

PAN-90806 (PanOptica) is a topical formulation of a small molecule, a tyrosine kinase inhibitor (TKI), to treat wet AMD. In phase 1/2 of a dose-ranging clinical trial, more than half of patients receiving PAN-90806 once a day for 12 weeks completed the study without needing anti-VEGF rescue therapy. Fourteen of the 51 patients in the study, 88% experienced clinical improvement of their condition or their disease's stability [55].

Squalamine lactate (Genaera Corporation) is an amino sterol derived from the dogfish shark's cartilage that blocks VEGF, PDGF basic fibroblast growth binding calmodulin and its chaperones. A phase 2 clinical trial showed improved vision when squalamine lactate was used in combination with anti-VEGF treatments [56, 57].

3.4 Extended-release options

The extended-release options may also reduce the burden of intravitreal injections.

The port delivery system (PDS; Hoffmann-La Roche) is a permanent, refillable implant, which is surgically placed at the pars plana through an incision in the sclera. PDS continuously releases concentrated ranibizumab by passive diffusion into the vitreous cavity.

Phase 2 of the LADDER clinical trial showed similar functional and anatomical outcomes after nine months of treatment with ranibizumab delivered through PDS or monthly intravitreal injections of ranibizumab [58, 59]. The mean time for the first PDS refill was 15 months, with 80% of patients not requiring a PDS refill for six or more months. Phase 3 of the ARCHWAY clinical trial is ongoing [60].

GB-102 (Graybug Vision) is a depot formulation of sunitinib malate that might need only 2 or 3 treatments per year [61]. Phase 2 of the ALTISSIMO clinical trial evaluated the safety and effect duration of GB-102 intravitreal injections administered every six months compared to aflibercept intravitreal injections administered every two months [62]. The results are currently pending.

NT-503 (Neurotech Pharmaceuticals) is a biological sustained drug delivery device that can provide anti-VEGF therapy's continuous delivery. Preliminary studies show that the device can be implanted safely in humans [63]. The results of phases 1 and 2 of clinical trials are pending [64].

Aflibercept Hydrogel Depot (Regeneron Pharmaceuticals and Ocular Therapeutix™) is a delivery system based on a PolyActive hydrogel copolymer's microparticles. In studies with animals intravitreally injected with aflibercept hydrogel depot a, sustained and controlled release of aflibercept was achieved. No adverse effects in the eyes of healthy rhesus macaques were observed for up to 6 months [65].

pSivida Durasert Technology (EyePoint Pharmaceuticals, Inc.) can be used to deliver different drugs for extended periods (months or even years) with a single application. Delivery of a tyrosine kinase inhibitor in animals provided promising results [66].

3.5 Gene therapy

Gene therapy is based on the insertion of an anti-VEGF coding sequence into retinal cells' DNA through a viral vector.

ADVM-022 (Adverum) produces an anti-VEGF-A fusion protein delivered through intravitreal injection via the AAV.7 m8 viral vector. Phase 1 of the OPTIC clinical trial showed that treatment with a single injection prevented additional anti-VEGF treatment over six months [67, 68].

RGX-314 (RegenexBio) (Rockville, MA, USA) produces an anti-VEGF A fab delivered through a subretinal treatment via an AAV8 viral vector. Phases 1/2a of the AAVIATE clinical trial showed a decrease in injection burden without significant inflammation or adverse effects [69]. Phase 2b of the AAVIATE clinical trial will explore a suprachoroidal injection [70].

Retinostat (Oxford BioMedica) is a lentiviral vector expressing endostatin and angiostatin to inhibit angiogenesis potentially. Phase 1 clinical trial showed that the LentiVector® gene therapy platform safely and efficiently delivered genes to the retina resulting in stable, long-term expression [71].

AAV2-sFLT01 (Genzyme, a Sanofi Company) is a vector that expresses a modified soluble Flt1 receptor designed to neutralize the proangiogenic activities of VEGF via an intravitreal injection. Phase 1 clinical trial showed that AAV2-sFLT01 was safe and that there was good tolerance to this vector [72]. After three years of follow-up, AAV2-sFLT01 appears to be generally safe, well-tolerated and does not appear to raise any new safety concerns [73].

AAVCAGsCD59 (Hemera Biosciences) is a molecule that targets the terminal step of complement activation that leads to the formation of the membrane attack complex. Two-phase 1 clinical trials for both exudative and dry AMD showed that subretinal injection of AAV-CD59 attenuated the formation of laser-induced choroidal neovascularization by around 60% in mice, even when the site of delivery was distal to the laser-induced choroidal neovascularization site [74].

An alternative for genetic interference is small interfering RNA (siRNA) that inhibits the protein-coding genes and prevent protein synthesis. Delivery can be by the topical installation or intravitreal injection. Bevasiranib (Opko) was the first siRNA used, but it did not show efficacy in phase 3 of the COBALT clinical trial [75]. AGN211745 (Alergan) was designed to reduce pathologic angiogenesis mediated by both VEGF *and* PIG. The study was terminated early due to a company decision (non-safety-related), and for this reason, certain outcome measures were not analyzed [76].

PF-655 (Pfizer) is a siRNA that inhibits expression of the hypoxia-inducible gene RTP801, which inhibits the mammalian target of the rapamycin (mTOR) signaling pathway and reduces VEGF-A production. Results from phase 2 of the MONET clinical trial showed that the combination of PF-655 with ranibizumab led to an average gain in visual acuity superior to the one observed for patients under ranibizumab monotherapy [77].

4. Conclusion

There are many potential therapeutic options for AMD. New treatment options for dry AMD that slow disease progression or re-establish retinal cells are becoming a reality. For wet AMD, new drugs that could lead to a longer half-life in the vitreous, lower costs, and more potent anti-angiogenesis activity, should be approved soon. With the increase of population longevity, AMD incidence and prevalence will most probably increase, and these therapies may reduce both the societal and individual treatment burden. Although they are in the earlier clinical trial phases, the authors consider that the cell-based therapies for dry AMD and gene therapy for wet AMD are the more promising therapies for the future because they tend to correct the source's problem. The new COVID vaccines also represent a significant step in this area, and these novel technologies may be future treatments for many other diseases.

Conflict of interest

The authors declare no conflict of interest.

Author details

Ana Marta[1,2*] and Bernardete Pessoa[1,2]

1 Centro Hospitalar Universitário do Porto (CHUP), Oporto, Portugal

2 Instituto Ciências Biomédicas Abel Salazar (ICBAS), Oporto, Portugal

*Address all correspondence to: analuisamarta2@gmail.com

IntechOpen

References

[1] Wong WL, Su X, Li X, Cheung CMG, Klein R, Cheng C-Y, et al. Global prevalence of age-related macular degeneration and disease burden projection for 2020 and 2040: a systematic review and meta-analysis. The Lancet Global Health. 2014 Feb 1;2(2):e106–e116.

[2] Al-Zamil WM, Yassin SA. Recent developments in age-related macular degeneration: a review. Clin Interv Aging. 2017;12:1313-1330.

[3] M G-M, P S-R, M F-R, Mj A, Mj R-C, M S-V, et al. Pharmacological Advances in the Treatment of Age-related Macular Degeneration. Curr Med Chem. 2020 Jan 1;27(4):583-598.

[4] Boyle J, Vukicevic M, Koklanis K, Itsiopoulos C, Rees G. Experiences of patients undergoing repeated intravitreal anti-vascular endothelial growth factor injections for neovascular age-related macular degeneration. Psychol Health Med. 2018 Feb;23(2):127-140.

[5] Prenner JL, Halperin LS, Rycroft C, Hogue S, Williams Liu Z, Seibert R. Disease Burden in the Treatment of Age-Related Macular Degeneration: Findings From a Time-and-Motion Study. Am J Ophthalmol. 2015 Oct;160(4):725-731.e1.

[6] Ciulla TA, Hussain RM, Pollack JS, Williams DF. Visual Acuity Outcomes and Anti-Vascular Endothelial Growth Factor Therapy Intensity in Neovascular Age-Related Macular Degeneration Patients: A Real-World Analysis of 49 485 Eyes. Ophthalmol Retina. 2020 Jan;4(1):19-30.

[7] Rofagha S, Bhisitkul RB, Boyer DS, Sadda SR, Zhang K, SEVEN-UP Study Group. Seven-year outcomes in ranibizumab-treated patients in ANCHOR, MARINA, and HORIZON: a multicenter cohort study (SEVEN-UP). Ophthalmology. 2013 Nov;120(11): 2292-2299.

[8] Holz FG, Sadda SR, Busbee B, Chew EY, Mitchell P, Tufail A, et al. Efficacy and Safety of Lampalizumab for Geographic Atrophy Due to Age-Related Macular Degeneration: Chroma and Spectri Phase 3 Randomized Clinical Trials. JAMA Ophthalmol. 2018 Jun 1;136(6):666-677.

[9] Yehoshua Z, de Amorim Garcia Filho CA, Nunes RP, Gregori G, Penha FM, Moshfeghi AA, et al. Systemic complement inhibition with eculizumab for geographic atrophy in age-related macular degeneration: the COMPLETE study. Ophthalmology. 2014 Mar;121(3):693-701.

[10] Liao DS, Grossi FV, El Mehdi D, Gerber MR, Brown DM, Heier JS, et al. Complement C3 Inhibitor Pegcetacoplan for Geographic Atrophy Secondary to Age-Related Macular Degeneration: A Randomized Phase 2 Trial. Ophthalmology. 2020 Feb 1;127(2):186-195.

[11] Apellis Pharmaceuticals, Inc. A Phase III, Multi-Center, Randomized, Double-Masked, Sham Controlled Study to Compare the Efficacy and Safety of Intravitreal APL-2 Therapy With Sham Injections in Patients With Geographic Atrophy (GA) Secondary to Age-Related Macular Degeneration (AMD) [Internet]. clinicaltrials.gov; 2020 Sep [cited 2021 Mar 29]. Report No.: NCT03525600. Available from: https:// clinicaltrials.gov/ct2/show/ NCT03525600

[12] Jaffe GJ, Westby K, Csaky KG, Monés J, Pearlman JA, Patel SS, et al. C5 Inhibitor Avacincaptad Pegol for Geographic Atrophy Due to Age-Related Macular Degeneration: A Randomized

Pivotal Phase 2/3 Trial. Ophthalmology. 2021 Apr;128(4):576-586.

[13] Chinskey ND, Besirli CG, Zacks DN. Retinal neuroprotection in dry age-related macular degeneration. Drug Discovery Today: Therapeutic Strategies. 2013 Mar 1;10(1):e21–e24.

[14] Allingham MJ, Mettu PS, Cousins SW. Elamipretide, a Mitochondrial-Targeted Drug, for the Treatment of Vision Loss in Dry AMD with High Risk Drusen: Results of the Phase 1 ReCLAIM Study. Invest Ophthalmol Vis Sci. 2019 Jul 22;60(9):361-361.

[15] Stealth BioTherapeutics Inc. A Phase 2 Randomized, Double-Masked, Placebo-Controlled Clinical Study to Evaluate the Safety, Efficacy and Pharmacokinetics of Elamipretide in Subjects With Age-Related Macular Degeneration With Non-central Geographic Atrophy [Internet]. clinicaltrials.gov; 2021 Feb [cited 2021 Mar 29]. Report No.: NCT03891875. Available from: https://clinicaltrials. gov/ct2/show/NCT03891875

[16] Retinal Physician - Brimonidine Drug Delivery System for Geographic Atrophy [Internet]. Retinal Physician. [cited 2021 Mar 31]. Available from: https://www.retinalphysician.com/ issues/2019/november-2019/ brimonidine-drug-delivery-system-for-geographic-at

[17] Allergan. Safety and Efficacy of Brimonidine Posterior Segment Drug Delivery System in Patients With Geographic Atrophy Secondary to Age-related Macular Degeneration [Internet]. clinicaltrials.gov; 2019 Mar [cited 2021 Mar 29]. Report No.: NCT02087085. Available from: https:// clinicaltrials.gov/ct2/show/ NCT02087085

[18] A Phase 2a clinical trial of ALK-001 in geographic atrophy - Leonide Saad [Internet]. [cited 2021 Mar 31]. Available from: https://grantome.com/ grant/NIH/R44-EY021988-02A1

[19] Alkeus Pharmaceuticals, Inc. A Phase 2/3 Multicenter, Randomized, Double-masked, Parallel-group, Placebo-controlled Study to Investigate the Safety, Pharmacokinetics, Tolerability, and Efficacy of ALK-001 in Geographic Atrophy Secondary to Age-related Macular Degeneration [Internet]. clinicaltrials.gov; 2020 Jul [cited 2021 Mar 29]. Report No.: NCT03845582. Available from: https:// clinicaltrials.gov/ct2/show/ NCT03845582

[20] Ammar MJ, Hsu J, Chiang A, Ho AC, Regillo CD. Age-related macular degeneration therapy: a review. Curr Opin Ophthalmol. 2020 May;31(3):215-221.

[21] Song WK, Park K-M, Kim H-J, Lee JH, Choi J, Chong SY, et al. Treatment of Macular Degeneration Using Embryonic Stem Cell-Derived Retinal Pigment Epithelium: Preliminary Results in Asian Patients. Stem Cell Reports. 2015 Apr 30;4(5):860-872.

[22] Qiu TG. Transplantation of human embryonic stem cell-derived retinal pigment epithelial cells (MA09-hRPE) in macular degeneration. npj Regenerative Medicine. 2019 Aug 27;4(1):1-5.

[23] Astellas Institute for Regenerative Medicine. A Phase I/II, Open-Label, Multi-Center, Prospective Study to Determine the Safety and Tolerability of Sub-retinal Transplantation of Human Embryonic Stem Cell Derived Retinal Pigmented Epithelial (MA09-hRPE) Cells in Patients With Advanced Dry AMD [Internet]. clinicaltrials.gov; 2017 Feb [cited 2021 Mar 29]. Report No.: NCT01344993. Available from: https:// clinicaltrials.gov/ct2/show/ NCT01344993

[24] Koss MJ, Falabella P, Stefanini FR, Pfister M, Thomas BB, Kashani AH, et al. Subretinal implantation of a monolayer of human embryonic stem cell-derived retinal pigment epithelium: a feasibility and safety study in Yucatán minipigs. Graefes Arch Clin Exp Ophthalmol. 2016 Aug;254(8):1553-1565.

[25] Kashani AH, Lebkowski JS, Rahhal FM, Avery RL, Salehi-Had H, Dang W, et al. A bioengineered retinal pigment epithelial monolayer for advanced, dry age-related macular degeneration. Sci Transl Med. 2018 Apr 4;10(435).

[26] Regenerative Patch Technologies, LLC. A Phase I/IIa Safety Study of Subretinal Implantation of CPCB-RPE1 (Human Embryonic Stem Cell-Derived Retinal Pigment Epithelial Cells Seeded on a Polymeric Substrate) in Subjects With Advanced, Dry Age-Related Macular Degeneration (AMD) [Internet]. clinicaltrials.gov; 2020 May [cited 2021 Mar 29]. Report No.: NCT02590692. Available from: https://clinicaltrials.gov/ct2/show/NCT02590692

[27] Wang Y, Wang VM, Chan C-C. The role of anti-inflammatory agents in age-related macular degeneration (AMD) treatment. Eye. 2011 Feb;25(2):127-139.

[28] PhD PY MD. A Randomized, Double Blind, Placebo Controlled Study Evaluating ORACEA® in Subjects With Geographic Atrophy Secondary to Non-Exudative Age-Related Macular Degeneration [Internet]. clinicaltrials.gov; 2018 Oct [cited 2021 Mar 29]. Report No.: study/NCT01782989. Available from: https://clinicaltrials.gov/ct2/show/study/NCT01782989

[29] Genentech, Inc. A Phase II, Multicenter, Randomized, Single-Masked, Sham-Controlled Study to Assess Safety, Tolerability, and Efficacy of Intravitreal Injections of FHTR2163 in Patients With Geographic Atrophy Secondary to Age-Related Macular Degeneration (GALLEGO) [Internet]. clinicaltrials.gov; 2021 Mar [cited 2021 Mar 29]. Report No.: NCT03972709. Available from: https://clinicaltrials.gov/ct2/show/NCT03972709

[30] Dugel PU, Koh A, Ogura Y, Jaffe GJ, Schmidt-Erfurth U, Brown DM, et al. HAWK and HARRIER: Phase 3, Multicenter, Randomized, Double-Masked Trials of Brolucizumab for Neovascular Age-Related Macular Degeneration. Ophthalmology. 2020 Jan 1;127(1):72-84.

[31] Allergan. Safety and Efficacy of Abicipar Pegol (AGN-150998) in Patients With Neovascular Age-related Macular Degeneration (SEQUOIA Study) [Internet]. clinicaltrials.gov; 2020 Jul [cited 2021 Mar 28]. Report No.: NCT02462486. Available from: https://clinicaltrials.gov/ct2/show/NCT02462486

[32] Allergan. Safety and Efficacy of Abicipar Pegol (AGN-150998) in Patients With Neovascular Age-related Macular Degeneration (CEDAR Study) [Internet]. clinicaltrials.gov; 2020 Jul [cited 2021 Mar 28]. Report No.: NCT02462928. Available from: https://clinicaltrials.gov/ct2/show/NCT02462928

[33] Kunimoto D, Yoon YH, Wykoff CC, Chang A, Khurana RN, Maturi RK, et al. Efficacy and Safety of Abicipar in Neovascular Age-Related Macular Degeneration: 52-Week Results of Phase 3 Randomized Controlled Study. Ophthalmology. 2020 Oct 1;127(10):1331-1344.

[34] Hussain RM, Weng CY, Wykoff CC, Gandhi RA, Hariprasad SM. Abicipar pegol for neovascular age-related macular degeneration. Expert Opin Biol Ther. 2020 Sep;20(9):999-1008.

[35] Li X, Xu G, Wang Y, Xu X, Liu X, Tang S, et al. Safety and efficacy of conbercept in neovascular age-related macular degeneration: results from a 12-month randomized phase 2 study: AURORA study. Ophthalmology. 2014 Sep;121(9):1740-1747.

[36] Liu K, Song Y, Xu G, Ye J, Wu Z, Liu X, et al. Conbercept for Treatment of Neovascular Age-related Macular Degeneration: Results of the Randomized Phase 3 PHOENIX Study. Am J Ophthalmol. 2019 Jan;197:156-167.

[37] Chengdu Kanghong Biotech Co., Ltd. A Multicenter, Double-Masked, Randomized, Dose-Ranging Trial to Evaluate the Efficacy and Safety of Conbercept Intravitreal Injection in Subjects With Neovascular Age-Related Macular Degeneration (AMD) (PANDA-2) [Internet]. clinicaltrials. gov; 2020 Oct [cited 2021 Mar 28]. Report No.: NCT03630952. Available from: https://clinicaltrials.gov/ct2/ show/NCT03630952

[38] Chengdu Kanghong Biotech Co., Ltd. A Multicenter, Double-Masked, Randomized, Dose-Ranging Trial to Evaluate the Efficacy and Safety of Conbercept Intravitreal Injection in Subjects With Neovascular Age-Related Macular Degeneration (AMD) (PANDA-1) [Internet]. clinicaltrials. gov; 2020 Oct [cited 2021 Mar 28]. Report No.: NCT03577899. Available from: https://clinicaltrials.gov/ct2/ show/NCT03577899

[39] Opthea Limited. A Dose-Ranging Study of Intravitreal OPT-302 in Combination With Ranibizumab, Compared With Ranibizumab Alone, in Participants With Neovascular Age-Related Macular Degeneration (Wet AMD) [Internet]. clinicaltrials.gov; 2021 Jan [cited 2021 Mar 29]. Report No.: NCT03345082. Available from: https://clinicaltrials.gov/ct2/show/ NCT03345082

[40] Dugel PU, Boyer DS, Antoszyk AN, Steinle NC, Varenhorst MP, Pearlman JA, et al. Phase 1 Study of OPT-302 Inhibition of Vascular Endothelial Growth Factors C and D for Neovascular Age-Related Macular Degeneration. Ophthalmol Retina. 2020 Mar;4(3):250-263.

[41] Opthea Limited. A Phase 3, Multicentre, Double-masked, Randomised Study to Evaluate the Efficacy and Safety of Intravitreal OPT-302 in Combination With Ranibizumab, Compared With Ranibizumab Alone, in Participants With nAMD [Internet]. clinicaltrials. gov; 2021 Feb [cited 2021 Mar 29]. Report No.: NCT04757610. Available from: https://clinicaltrials.gov/ct2/ show/NCT04757610

[42] Danzig C, Quezada C, Basu K, Grzeschik S, Sahni J, Silverman D, et al. Efficacy and safety of faricimab every 16 or 12 weeks for neovascular age-related macular degeneration: STAIRWAY phase 2 results. Invest Ophthalmol Vis Sci. 2019 Jul 22;60(9):1212-1212.

[43] Hoffmann-La Roche. STAIRWAY: Simultaneous Blockade of Angiopoietin-2 and VEGF-A With the Bispecific Antibody RO6867461 (RG7716) for Extended Durability in the Treatment of Neovascular Age-Related Macular Degeneration [Internet]. clinicaltrials.gov; 2020 Dec [cited 2021 Mar 26]. Report No.: NCT03038880. Available from: https:// clinicaltrials.gov/ct2/show/ NCT03038880

[44] Hoffmann-La Roche. A Phase III, Multicenter, Randomized, Double-Masked, Active Comparator-Controlled Study to Evaluate the Efficacy and Safety of Faricimab in Patients With Neovascular Age-Related Macular Degeneration (TENAYA) [Internet]. clinicaltrials.gov; 2021 Mar [cited 2021 Mar 26]. Report No.: NCT03823287.

Available from: https://clinicaltrials.gov/ct2/show/NCT03823287

[45] Hoffmann-La Roche. A Phase III, Multicenter, Randomized, Double-Masked, Active Comparator-Controlled Study to Evaluate the Efficacy and Safety of Faricimab in Patients With Neovascular Age-Related Macular Degeneration (LUCERNE) [Internet]. clinicaltrials.gov; 2021 Mar [cited 2021 Mar 26]. Report No.: NCT03823300. Available from: https://clinicaltrials.gov/ct2/show/NCT03823300

[46] KSI-301 for exudative retinal disease showing safety, efficacy, and durability [Internet]. Modern Retina. [cited 2021 Mar 30]. Available from: https://www.modernretina.com/view/ksi-301-for-exudative-retinal-disease-showing-safety-efficacy-and-durability

[47] Kodiak Sciences Inc. A Phase 2b/3, Prospective, Randomized, Double-masked, Active Comparator-controlled, Multi-center Study to Investigate the Efficacy and Safety of Repeated Intravitreal Administration of KSI-301 in Subjects With Neovascular (Wet) Age-related Macular Degeneration. [Internet]. clinicaltrials.gov; 2020 Nov [cited 2021 Mar 29]. Report No.: NCT04049266. Available from: https://clinicaltrials.gov/ct2/show/NCT04049266

[48] Outlook Therapeutics, Inc. A Clinical Effectiveness, Multicenter, Randomized, Double-masked, Controlled Study of the Efficacy and Safety of ONS-5010 in Subjects With Subfoveal Choroidal Neovascularization (CNV) Secondary to Age-related Macular Degeneration [Internet]. clinicaltrials.gov; 2020 Sep [cited 2021 Mar 28]. Report No.: NCT03844074. Available from: https://clinicaltrials.gov/ct2/show/NCT03844074

[49] Bioeq GmbH. Efficacy and Safety of the Biosimilar Ranibizumab FYB201 in Comparison to Lucentis in Patients With Neovascular Age-related Macular Degeneration [Internet]. clinicaltrials.gov; 2019 Jan [cited 2021 Mar 28]. Report No.: NCT02611778. Available from: https://clinicaltrials.gov/ct2/show/NCT02611778

[50] Samsung Bioepis Co., Ltd. A Phase III Randomised, Double-masked, Parallel Group, Multicentre Study to Compare the Efficacy, Safety, Pharmacokinetics and Immunogenicity Between SB11 and Lucentis® in Subjects With Neovascular Age-related Macular Degeneration [Internet]. clinicaltrials.gov; 2020 Jun [cited 2021 Mar 28]. Report No.: NCT03150589. Available from: https://clinicaltrials.gov/ct2/show/NCT03150589

[51] Xbrane Biopharma AB. A Phase III Double-Blind, Parallel Group, Multicenter Study to Compare the Efficacy and Safety of Xlucane Versus Lucentis® in Patients With Neovascular Age-Related Macular Degeneration [Internet]. clinicaltrials.gov; 2020 Jun [cited 2021 Mar 28]. Report No.: NCT03805100. Available from: https://clinicaltrials.gov/ct2/show/NCT03805100

[52] Joussen AM, Wolf S, Kaiser PK, Boyer D, Schmelter T, Sandbrink R, et al. The Developing Regorafenib Eye drops for neovascular Age-related Macular degeneration (DREAM) study: an open-label phase II trial. Br J Clin Pharmacol. 2019 Feb;85(2):347-355.

[53] Csaky KG, Dugel PU, Pierce AJ, Fries MA, Kelly DS, Danis RP, et al. Clinical evaluation of pazopanib eye drops versus ranibizumab intravitreal injections in subjects with neovascular age-related macular degeneration. Ophthalmology. 2015 Mar;122(3):579-588.

[54] Poor SH, Adams CM, Ferriere M, Weichselberger A, Grosskreutz CL, Weissgerber G. Topical VEGF receptor

inhibitor, LHA510, did not demonstrate efficacy in a Proof-of-Concept study in patients with neovascular age-related macular degeneration (nv AMD). Invest Ophthalmol Vis Sci. 2018 Jul 13;59(9):2394-2394.

[55] PanOptica, Inc. A Randomized, Double Masked, Uncontrolled, Multicenter Phase I/II Study to Evaluate Safety and Tolerability of PAN-90806 Eye Drops, Suspension in Treatment-Naïve Participants With Neovascular Age-Related Macular Degeneration (AMD) [Internet]. clinicaltrials.gov; 2019 Jul [cited 2021 Mar 29]. Report No.: NCT03479372. Available from: https://clinicaltrials.gov/ct2/show/NCT03479372

[56] Slakter JS, Ciulla TA, Elman MJ, Singerman LJ, Stoller G, Kaiser PK, et al. Final Results from a Phase 2 Study of Squalamine Lactate Ophthalmic Solution 0.2% (OHR-102) in the Treatment of Neovascular Age-related Macular Degeneration (AMD). Invest Ophthalmol Vis Sci. 2015 Jun 11;56(7):4805-4805.

[57] Ohr Pharmaceutical Inc. Phase II Study of the Efficacy and Safety of Squalamine Lactate Ophthalmic Formulation 0.2% BID in Subjects With Neovascular AMD. [Internet]. clinicaltrials.gov; 2015 Jun [cited 2021 Mar 29]. Report No.: NCT01678963. Available from: https://clinicaltrials.gov/ct2/show/NCT01678963

[58] Genentech, Inc. A Phase II, Multicenter, Randomized, Active Treatment-Controlled Study of the Efficacy and Safety of the Ranibizumab Port Delivery System for Sustained Delivery of Ranibizumab in Patients With Subfoveal Neovascular Age-Related Macular Degeneration [Internet]. clinicaltrials.gov; 2019 Jun [cited 2021 Mar 28]. Report No.: NCT02510794. Available from: https://clinicaltrials.gov/ct2/show/NCT02510794

[59] Campochiaro PA, Marcus DM, Awh CC, Regillo C, Adamis AP, Bantseev V, et al. The Port Delivery System with Ranibizumab for Neovascular Age-Related Macular Degeneration: Results from the Randomized Phase 2 Ladder Clinical Trial. Ophthalmology. 2019 Aug;126(8):1141-1154.

[60] Hoffmann-La Roche. Phase III, Multicenter, Randomized, Visual Assessor-Masked, Active-Comparator Study of the Efficacy, Safety, and Pharmacokinetics of the Port Delivery System With Ranibizumab in Patients With Neovascular Age-Related Macular Degeneration [Internet]. clinicaltrials.gov; 2021 Mar [cited 2021 Mar 28]. Report No.: NCT03677934. Available from: https://clinicaltrials.gov/ct2/show/NCT03677934

[61] GB-102 for Wet AMD: A Novel Injectable Formulation that Safely Delivers Active Levels of Sunitinib to the Retina and RPE/Choroid for Over Four Months | IOVS | ARVO Journals [Internet]. [cited 2021 Mar 30]. Available from: https://iovs.arvojournals.org/article.aspx?articleid=2563200

[62] Graybug Vision. A Phase 2b Multicenter Dose-Ranging Study Evaluating the Safety and Efficacy of Sunitinib Malate Depot Formulation (GB-102) Compared to Aflibercept in Subjects With Neovascular (Wet) Age-related Macular Degeneration (ALTISSIMO Study) [Internet]. clinicaltrials.gov; 2021 Jan [cited 2021 Mar 29]. Report No.: NCT03953079. Available from: https://clinicaltrials.gov/ct2/show/NCT03953079

[63] Guerrero-Naranjo JL, Quiroz-Mercado H, Sanchez-Bermudez G, Schoonewolff F, Longoria SS, Vera RR, et al. Safety of implantation of the NT-503 device in patients with Choroidal Neovascularization secondary to

Age-related Macular Degeneration. Invest Ophthalmol Vis Sci. 2013 Jun 16;54(15):3298-3298.

[64] Neurotech Pharmaceuticals. A Multi-Center, Two-Stage, Open-Label Phase I and Randomized, Active Controlled, Masked Phase II Study to Evaluate the Safety and Efficacy of Intravitreal Implantation of NT-503-3 Encapsulated Cell Technology Compared With Eylea for the Treatment of Recurrent CNV Secondary to AMD [Internet]. clinicaltrials.gov; 2016 Nov [cited 2021 Mar 29]. Report No.: study/ NCT02228304. Available from: https:// clinicaltrials.gov/ct2/show/study/ NCT02228304

[65] Kim S, Kang-Mieler JJ, Liu W, Wang Z, Yiu G, Teixeira LBC, et al. Safety and Biocompatibility of Aflibercept-Loaded Microsphere Thermo-Responsive Hydrogel Drug Delivery System in a Nonhuman Primate Model. Transl Vis Sci Technol [Internet]. [cited 2021 Mar 30];9(3). Available from: https://www.ncbi.nlm. nih.gov/pmc/articles/PMC7354880/

[66] Preclinical studies show pSivida's Durasert implant delivering TKI just as effective as injection of FDA-approved biologic in wet AMD; shares up 5% (NASDAQ:EYPT) [Internet]. SeekingAlpha. [cited 2021 Mar 30]. Available from: https://seekingalpha. com/news/3191730-preclinical- studies-show-psividas-durasert- implant-delivering-tki-just-effective- injection-of

[67] Adverum Biotechnologies, Inc. An Open Label Phase 1 Study of ADVM-022 (AAV.7m8-aflibercept) in Neovascular (Wet) Age-Related Macular Degeneration [Internet]. clinicaltrials. gov; 2020 Nov [cited 2021 Mar 28]. Report No.: NCT03748784. Available from: https://clinicaltrials.gov/ct2/ show/NCT03748784

[68] http://fyra.io. Intravitreal In-Office Anti-VEGF Gene Therapy [Internet]. Retina Today. Bryn Mawr Communications; [cited 2021 Mar 30]. Available from: https://retinatoday.com/ articles/2019-nov-dec/ intravitreal-in-office-anti-vegf- gene-therapy

[69] Regenxbio Inc. A Phase I/IIa, Open-label, Multiple-cohort, Dose- escalation Study to Evaluate the Safety and Tolerability of Gene Therapy With RGX-314 in Subjects With Neovascular AMD (nAMD) [Internet]. clinicaltrials. gov; 2020 Oct [cited 2021 Mar 28]. Report No.: NCT03066258. Available from: https://clinicaltrials.gov/ct2/ show/NCT03066258

[70] Regenxbio Inc. A Phase 2, Randomized, Dose-escalation, Ranibizumab-controlled Study to Evaluate the Efficacy, Safety, and Tolerability of RGX-314 Gene Therapy Delivered Via One or Two Suprachoroidal Space (SCS) Injections in Participants With Neovascular Age-Related Macular Degeneration (nAMD) (AAVIATE) [Internet]. clinicaltrials.gov; 2020 Aug [cited 2021 Mar 28]. Report No.: NCT04514653. Available from: https://clinicaltrials. gov/ct2/show/NCT04514653

[71] Lauer AK, Campochiaro PA, Sohn EH, Kelleher M, Harrop R, Loader J, et al. Phase I Safety and Tolerability results for RetinoStat®, a Lentiviral Vector Expressing Endostatin and Angiostatin, in Patients with Advanced Neovascular Age-Related Macular Degeneration. Invest Ophthalmol Vis Sci [Internet]. 2016 Sep 26 [cited 2021 Mar 30];57(12). Available from: https://iovs.arvojournals.org/ article.aspx?articleid=2562864

[72] Heier JS, Kherani S, Desai S, Dugel P, Kaushal S, Cheng SH, et al. Intravitreous injection of AAV2-sFLT01 in patients with advanced neovascular age-related macular degeneration: a phase 1, open-label trial. The Lancet. 2017 Jul 1;390(10089):50-61.

[73] Varona R, Le-Halpere A, Campochiaro PA, Heier J, Dugel PU, Barsamian M, et al. 3-Year Interim Safety Profile of Adeno-Associated Virus Serotype 2-soluble Variant of the Vascular Endothelial Growth Factor Receptor Type 1 (AAV2-sFLT01) Administered by Intravitreal Injection in Patients with Neovascular Age-Related Macular Degeneration. Invest Ophthalmol Vis Sci. 2017 Jun 23;58(8):2321-2321.

[74] Cashman SM, Ramo K, Kumar-Singh R. A Non Membrane-Targeted Human Soluble CD59 Attenuates Choroidal Neovascularization in a Model of Age Related Macular Degeneration. PLoS One [Internet]. 2011 Apr 28 [cited 2021 Mar 30];6(4). Available from: https://www.ncbi.nlm.nih.gov/pmc/articles/PMC3084256/

[75] OPKO Health, Inc. A Phase 3, Randomized, Double-masked, Parallel-assignment Study of Intravitreal Bevasiranib Sodium, Administered Every 8 or 12 Weeks as Maintenance Therapy Following Three Injections of Lucentis® Compared With Lucentis® Monotherapy Every 4 Weeks in Patients With Exudative Age-Related Macular Degeneration (AMD). [Internet]. clinicaltrials.gov; 2014 Sep [cited 2021 Mar 29]. Report No.: results/NCT00499590. Available from: https://clinicaltrials.gov/ct2/show/results/NCT00499590

[76] A Study Using Intravitreal Injections of a Small Interfering RNA in Patients With Age-Related Macular Degeneration - Full Text View - ClinicalTrials.gov [Internet]. [cited 2021 Mar 30]. Available from: https://clinicaltrials.gov/ct2/show/NCT00395057

[77] Nguyen QD, Schachar RA, Nduaka CI, Sperling M, Klamerus KJ, Chi-Burris K, et al. Evaluation of the siRNA PF-04523655 versus ranibizumab for the treatment of neovascular age-related macular degeneration (MONET Study). Ophthalmology. 2012 Sep;119(9):1867-1873.

Chapter 6

Saponin-Mediated Rejuvenation of Bruch's Membrane: A New Strategy for Intervention in Dry Age-Related Macular Degeneration (AMD)

Yunhee Lee, Eun Jung Ahn and Ali Hussain

Abstract

At present, there is no treatment modality for the vast majority of patients with dry AMD. The pathophysiology of AMD is complex but current evidence suggests that abnormal ageing of Bruch's membrane imparts a metabolic insult to the retinal pigment epithelium (RPE) and photoreceptor cells that leads eventually to the inflammatory-mediated death of these cells. Underlying mechanisms contributing to the pathology of Bruch's membrane include the accumulation of 'debris' and malfunction of the matrix metalloproteinase (MMP) system resulting in diminished metabolic support of the retina and inefficient removal of toxic pro-inflammatory mediators. Saponins are amphipathic molecules that have a hydrophobic tri-terpenoid lipid region and hydrophilic glycosidic chains that allow for the dispersion of these deposits in Bruch's and re-activation of the MMP system leading to a 2-fold improvement in the transport properties of the membrane. Such an intervention is expected to improve the bi-directional exchange of nutrients and waste products, thereby slowing the progression of dry AMD. This will be the first drug-based interventionist possibility to address dry AMD.

Keywords: macular degeneration, Bruch's membrane, extracellular matrix, ageing, saponins

1. Introduction

Blindness due to AMD is of great concern to the ageing elderly population since the prevalence of the disease in Europe, in those aged 60 years and over has been estimated to be 27.7% with a projected increase in numbers from 67 to 77 million by 2050 [1]. Clinically, AMD is broadly divided into early, intermediate and late (or advanced) forms. Early AMD is characterised by the presence of large drusen and pigmentary abnormalities such as hypo- or hyperpigmentation of the fundus. Progression to the late form results in geographic atrophy of the RPE followed by photoreceptor degeneration, known as 'dry' AMD. The late phase is also associated with secondary complications of neovascular episodes (comprising 10-20% patients), these being designated as 'wet' AMD.

The wet form of the disease can lead to rapid visual loss and considerable efforts at intervention have resulted in anti-vascular endothelial growth factor (anti-VEGF) intra-vitreal injections with a considerable degree of success in managing the neovascularisation, but the underlying progression of the disease is not altered. Thus, the vast majority of AMD patients (falling in the 'dry' AMD category) still await the development of a suitable treatment modality that can either slow or arrest the progression of the disease [2, 3].

The pathophysiology of AMD is highly complex due to the diverse genetic associations and considerable gene-environmental interactions exacerbated by the additional association of dietary and cardiovascular risk factors [4–6]. Furthermore, all these factors are superimposed on the normal ageing changes in the visual unit making it very difficult to nominate specific targets for intervention. Since age is the highest risk factor for the development of AMD, an understanding of the inherent stresses in the visual system would allow us to predict the likely effect of additional risk factors providing a more targeted approach towards therapy.

Briefly, in the visual unit, the photoreceptor is the primary site of sustained damage producing highly toxic compounds that can trigger an inflammatory response. However, this damage is rapidly transferred to the RPE by the daily shedding of outer segment discs and phagocytosis. Since the RPE also operates in the same oxidative environment as the photoreceptor cell, the engulfed discs undergo further damage resulting in compromised lysosomal degradation. Non-degradable material, comprising mainly lipofuscin-related products is either packaged and stored in the RPE or extruded as membraneous debris onto Bruch's membrane. With age, this debris accumulates in Bruch's compromising its ability to transport nutrients, anti-oxidants, and vitamins essential for RPE and photoreceptor function. The toxic metabolites in Bruch's are pro-inflammatory mediators and in the normal elderly, lead to a low-grade inflammatory response [7]. In advanced ageing associated with AMD, a chronic inflammatory response is precipitated leading to the death of RPE and photoreceptors.

For therapeutic intervention to be effective, the functional aspects of the RPE and Bruch's membrane need to be restored. We will examine the compositional and functional alterations of ageing RPE and Bruch's membrane, nominate suitable targets for intervention, and assess the potential for amphipathic saponin molecules to reverse these ageing changes as a potential therapy for dry AMD.

2. Underlying stresses in the visual unit leading to ageing and pathophysiology

Photoreceptor physiology is dependent on the supportive roles provided by the RPE and Bruch's membrane. Inherent stresses in these compartments lead to morphological and functional deterioration manifesting as 'normal' ageing changes but in the advanced ageing scenario of AMD culminate in the transition to pathology. The stresses within each compartment of the visual unit will be identified, providing therapeutic targets for intervention.

2.1 Stresses generated in photoreceptor cells

The photoreceptor is a highly specialised neuronal cell capable of detecting a single photon of light. Absorption of light by rhodopsin (R) present in the outer segment disc membranes leads to isomerization of the 11-cis retinal chromophore to its all-trans form (AT-RL), producing activated rhodopsin (R*). Amplification of the light signal begins by rapid lateral diffusion of R* over the disc membrane and interaction with many transducin molecules. Such high mobility of R* requires a very fluid membrane conferred by the high level of unsaturated docosahexanoic acid (DHA) in its membrane phospholipids. Further enzymatic amplification of the light signal by the guanalate cyclase-phosphodiesterase system leads to closure of sodium channels in the outer segment membrane resulting in hyper-polarisation of the cell and concomitant modulation of transmitter release. To meet the energy demands of these processes, the photoreceptor maintains the highest rates of oxidative metabolism of any cell in the body. Associated with this activity is the release of damaging oxygen radicals by the mitochondrial electron transport chain.

The presence of toxic retinoids, highly unsaturated fatty acids, high oxygen tension, high oxidative metabolism, and light is an explosive mixture for the generation of free-radical mediated damage. Since released AT-RL is highly toxic, it is rapidly reduced to all-trans retinol. However, AT-RL can react with phosphatidylethanol-amine to form retinylidene-phosphatidylethanolamine (NRPE) [8]. NRPE can react with a second molecule of AT-RL to form a bis-retinoid. Further modifications produce a variety of all-trans retinal dimers including A2E, the auto-fluorescent fluorophore of lipofuscin [9]. These bis-retinoids can undergo photo-oxidation to form oxo-aldehydes which then react with proteins to form advanced glycation end-products (AGEs) that are triggers of inflammatory processes [10].

Peroxidation of polyunsaturated fatty acids such as DHA results in fragmentation of the molecule leading to a mixture of compounds that bind to proteins [11, 12]. Oxidation of DHA produces carboxy-ethyl-pyrrole (CEP)-protein adducts. Thus, oxidation of PUFAs results in lipid aggregates, lipid-protein complexes, protein cross-link formation and CEP-adducts. These CEP-adducts have been localised to the RPE and drusen and being strongly immunogenic, activate the immune system [13].

Some protection from oxidative damage is afforded by the impressive anti-oxidant machinery (vitamins C&E, macular pigments, and enzymes such as catalase, peroxidase, and superoxide dismutase) [14, 15]. However, this protection in photoreceptors is dependent on an adequate supply of anti-oxidants and essential metals for the enzymic system by the RPE and Bruch's membrane. Despite these protective mechanisms, considerable damage is sustained by photoreceptors. Fortunately for the photoreceptor, this damage is confined to the outer segment discs and transferred to the RPE.

Therapeutic intervention to combat this damage has been considered resulting in the Age-Related Eye Disease Study (AREDS) vitamin and anti-oxidant supplements and their effectiveness will be discussed later.

2.2 Oxidative damage in the RPE

The RPE operates in the same oxidative environment as the photoreceptor cell and therefore, the toxic reactions initiated in the outer segments will continue in the phagolysosome. Lysosomal enzymes hydrolyse the normal, undamaged protein and lipid components. recycling the base metabolites back to the photoreceptor cell. Damaged proteins, lipid-derived adducts, protein cross-links due to lipid-carbonyl attack, and aggregated lipid complexes that are no longer susceptible to lysosomal enzymes remain in the phago-lysosomal sac [16]. The lysosomal hydrolysis of bis-retinoids results in the formation of the primary age pigment, A2E. A2E and other bis-retinoids undergo further oxidation to produce a variety of toxic products that not only damage lysosomal enzymes but also damage the lysosomal membrane inhibiting the proton pumps with the subsequent increase in pH that will further diminish lysosomal enzyme activity [17].

Un-hydrolysed lipoprotein and aggregated protein complexes together with bis-retinoids are packaged and stored as the auto-fluorescent pigment lipofuscin in membrane enclosed sacs. Lipofuscin content of the RPE increases with age and can amount to nearly 20% of cytoplasmic volume in the elderly [18]. Increased oxidative stress is inferred from the accumulation of AGEs in both ageing RPE and Bruch's membrane [19]. The RPE has a battery of anti-oxidants and a robust enzymic machinery to neutralise the oxidative stress and again, the components of the protective machinery are supplied by transport across Bruch's membrane. However, the age-related accumulation of bis-retinoids and damaged proteins suggests that the anti-oxidant system is not effective in tackling this threat.

The primary functions of the RPE are (a) phagocytosis of shed outer segment discs and their degradation, (b) vectorial transport of nutrients, lipids, metals, vitamins and anti-oxidants, and the removal of waste products generated in the photoreceptor cell, and (c) fluid transport from the sub-retinal space to the choroid. The effect of the age on the various functional parameters of the RPE are poorly understood. One report has suggested that phagocytic activity is halved between the ages of 30 and 80 years [20]. Another important function of the RPE is the delivery of nutrients, anti-oxidants, vitamins, etc supplied by the choroidal circulation to the photoreceptor cell. Since the RPE is the site of the outer blood-retinal barrier, all metabolites must cross the interior of the cell to gain access to photoreceptors. Therefore, transport across the RPE is mediated by passive diffusion or facilitated by active and passive carriers in the membrane. Most active carriers utilise the sodium electro-chemical gradient generated primarily by mitochondrial respiration [21]. However, A2E generated in the RPE binds to cytochrome C of the electron transport chain impairing mitochondrial respiration and this is expected to impact on the effectiveness of active carrier transport [22, 23].

There is little information of the effect of age on the activity of ligand carriers of the RPE due largely to interference from the adjacent Bruch's membrane. This is best illustrated with the transport of retinol (vitamin A). In elderly subjects and patients with early AMD, the recovery in dark-adaptation following a strong bleach is delayed [24, 25]. This delay is thought to be due to low levels of retinoids in the RPE and therefore slower transfer of 11-cis retinal to photoreceptors for regeneration of rhodopsin. Lowered levels of retinoids in the RPE could be due to lowered uptake by the RPE itself or diminished transport of retinol across Bruch's membrane. The fact that there is improvement in dark-adaptation following vitamin A supplementation would suggest inefficient delivery across Bruch's, rather than reduced uptake by the RPE as the contributary factor [26].

Fluid transport is another important function carried out by the RPE. Retinal fluids (originating from retinal capillary beds and retinal metabolism) are transported out by the RPE predominantly by an active process [27, 28]. The daily output of fluid from the RPE has been determined to be about 0.13 ± 0.11 μl/hour/mm^2 and metabolic insufficiency in the RPE would lead to fluids accumulating on top of the RPE resulting in macular oedema and/or retinal detachment [29, 30].

Therapeutic intervention in support of the RPE would require effective delivery of anti-oxidants and strengthening of its metabolic capability so as to reduce the generation of toxic products and assist in their rapid removal.

2.3 Compositional changes in ageing Bruch's membrane

Bruch's membrane mediates the exchange of nutrients and waste products between the choroidal blood supply and the RPE. An age-related compromise in these functions will reduce the capacity to supply essential nutrients to the RPE and photoreceptor cells increasing the risk of damage in these compartments.

The most obvious morphological change in Bruch's with age is increased thickness from about 1.5 μm in the young to 5.5 μm in the elderly [31]. This is due primarily to the deposition of normal and abnormal extracellular matrix (ECM) material. In the elderly, cross-linked and denatured (damaged) collagen accounts for nearly 50% of total collagen in Bruch's membrane [32]. There is also an increase in oxidative and non-enzymic glycosylation of proteins and lipids leading to the accumulation of toxic advanced glycation end-products, AGEs [33]. The membrane also shows an exponential increase in the level of lipid-rich debris [34]. Most of this debris arises from inefficient phagocytic processing of damaged outer segment discs in the RPE that is then extruded onto Bruch's membrane. This material then undergoes further oxidative modification with both the inherent matrix proteins and with passer-by constituents leading to further damage and deposition. Finally, the lipid components undergo free-energy driven aggregation leading to the accumulation of 100 nm diameter lipid-rich particles observed in the inner collagenous layer of Bruch's membrane [35].

Thus, in addition to the toxic metabolites mentioned above, deposits in Bruch's contain phospholipids, triglycerides, cholesterol, cholesterol esters, peroxidised lipids and apolipoproteins, immunoglobulins, amyloid, complement, and proteins specific to RPE function [36]. Heavy metal deposition has also been demonstrated that stabilises the debris in Bruch's [37].

The above changes result in gross morphological alteration of ageing Bruch's membrane that are expected to be detrimental to its transport functions (**Figure 1**).

Mechanisms exist to counteract the deleterious changes described above for Bruch's membrane. This involves the continuous synthesis and degradation of the extracellular matrix, the latter process being mediated by the matrix metalloproteinase (MMP) system [38]. Although this system performs well in the young, it deteriorates rapidly with age and more so in AMD [39].

2.4 Functional deterioration of ageing Bruch's membrane

Since Bruch's membrane is crucial for the exchange of nutrients and waste products, a deficiency in its transport functions will increase the risk of damage in the RPE and photoreceptor compartments for the reasons outlined earlier. The extent to which the compositional alterations of ageing Bruch's impact on its ability to remove

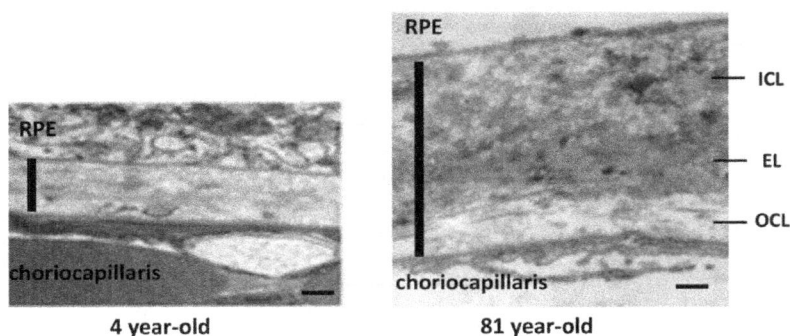

4 year-old   81 year-old

Figure 1.
Morphology of ageing Bruch's membrane. With age, Bruch's becomes thicker and contains a lot of debris rich in lipids, and abnormal matrix and non-matrix material. The increase in thickness alone will reduce the diffusional gradients for the transport of nutrients and waste products. Vertical bar denotes the thickness of Bruch's membrane. ICL, inner collagenous layer, EL, elastin layer; OC, outer collagenous layer. Bar marker: 1 μm.

fluids into the choroidal circulation, to supply adequate levels of essential nutrients, antioxidants, and vitamins to the RPE and photoreceptors, to maintain the rejuvenation potential of its membrane, and to modulate the occurrence of inflammatory responses will now be examined in both normal ageing and in the advanced ageing scenario of AMD.

2.4.1 Diminished fluid transport

The capacity for fluid transport across a membrane is designated by its hydraulic conductivity. As previously indicated, the daily output of fluid from the RPE and onto Bruch's membrane is about 0.13 ± 0.11 µl/hour/mm^2. To effectively transport this amount of fluid, Bruch's needs to have a minimum hydraulic conductivity of 0.65×10^{-10} m/s/Pa, and this level is referred to as the failure threshold [40, 41]. If hydraulic conductivity falls below this level, then fluid will accumulate on top of the membrane leading to a RPE detachment. Hydraulic conductivity of human Bruch's has been determined in 56 donors spanning the age range 1-91 years (**Figure 2**, modified from reference [40]). Conductivity was shown to decline exponentially with age and in the semi-log plot, the transformation is shown as a straight line. The half-life of the decay process was 16 years, i.e., conductivity was halved for every 16 years of life. Excess capacity is present in the younger population but with age, there is a drift towards the failure threshold. Extrapolating the straight line shows that the shelf-life of human Bruch's is about 123 years, but in the data of **Figure 2**, two of the normal donors have already reached the failure threshold. Bruch's from AMD donors showed a faster rate of decline in hydraulic conductivity [40] and as such, complications of RPE detachment are observed in about 12-20% of AMD patients [42].

For an effective therapeutic intervention in AMD, the exponential decay line in **Figure 2** needs to be elevated so as to avoid the failure threshold within the life-time of an individual.

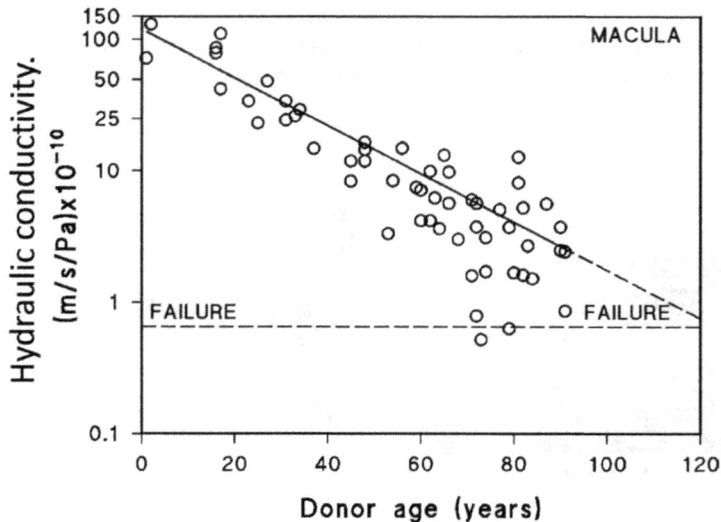

Figure 2.
Semi-logarithmic plot to show the exponential decay in the hydraulic conductivity of human Bruch's with age. (Modified from reference [40]).

2.4.2 Diminished metabolite and waste transport

Metabolites ranging from the simple sugars and amino acids to the much larger lipo-protein complexes are released from the fenestrated endothelium of the choriocapillaris vessels and traverse Bruch's by passive diffusion. Most of the essential metabolites such as heavy metals, vitamins (including vitamin A), and lipids are transported bound to carrier proteins that generally have a hydrodynamic radius of about 3-12 nm.

To assess the effect of age on the diffusional status of human Bruch's membrane, a FITC-albumin test probe was utilised that has a hydrodynamic radius of about 3.5 nm, similar to most carrier proteins. Diffusional experiments were conducted in standard Using chambers utilising isolated Bruch's membrane preparations from 33 donors, age range 12-92 years. The diffusional status of Bruch's membrane was observed to decrease exponentially with age, with a half-life of 18 years (**Figure 3**) [43]. Thus, over a human life-span, diffusional status was reduced by about 10-fold. We do not know the value of the failure threshold for diffusion across Bruch's membrane. However, since most elderly subjects show delayed dark-adaptation due to inefficient transport of vitamin A, the albumin diffusion values of subjects aged 77-87 years (0.024 nmol/6 mm/hour) were taken as the failure threshold.

Other in-vitro studies utilising serum proteins (MW 40-200 kDa) or FITC-dextran molecules (MW 21 kDA, radius 3.3 nm) have also shown a >10-fold reduction in diffusion capability over a human life-span [44, 45].

In AMD, the reduction in diffusional transport across Bruch's membrane was much more severe compared to age-matched controls [45]. This reduction in transport is expected to impact on the nutritional and anti-oxidant support of both RPE and photoreceptor cells, increasing oxidative stress. Similarly, transport in the opposite direction i.e., removal of toxic waste products from Bruch's membrane will also be diminished leading to greater oxidative modifications and generation of further toxic products.

As with hydraulic conductivity, for effective therapeutic intervention, the diffusional decay curves should be elevated away from the failure threshold.

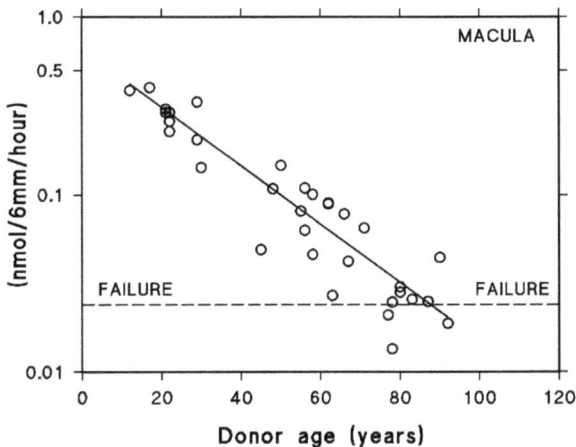

Figure 3.
The effect of age on the diffusion of albumin across human Bruch's. Semi-logarithmic plot showing the decay half-life to be 18 years.

Reduced diffusion within Bruch's membrane will also affect the protective mechanisms that depend on rapid mobility such as the interactions of complement factor H (CFH) with its many ligands and activation of pro-MMP2 in the regeneration of Bruch's. These aspects are described below.

2.4.3 Impaired regeneration in ageing Bruch's membrane

The ECM of Bruch's is continuously regenerated by coupled processes of synthesis and degradation. This ensures that damaged material is removed and replaced by new ECM components synthesised by the RPE, thereby maintaining the transport integrity of Bruch's membrane. Since abnormal collagen accumulates in ageing Bruch's (amounting to 50% of total collagen in the elderly), the regeneration process appears to be dysfunctional [32]. Little is known about the synthetic rate of ECM by the ageing RPE but the accumulation of damaged ECM components suggests problems with the degradation machinery.

Matrix degradation is mediated by a family of proteolytic enzymes called the matrix metalloproteinases (MMPs). These are synthesised in the RPE and released into Bruch's membrane as latent pro-enzymes (pro-MMPs) that on activation, following the removal of a small inhibitory peptide, can degrade almost all components of the ECM [38, 46]. In Bruch's, the major MMP species are pro-MMP2 and pro-MMP9, the former being the homeostatic enzyme in the system and the latter being the inducible form. Activation of pro-MMP2 occurs on the basolateral surface of the RPE by the initial formation of a binary complex between the membrane bound MMP-14 and the tissue inhibitor of MMPs, TIMP2. This then binds pro-MMP2 to form a tertiary complex that then results in the hydrolysis of the inhibitory peptide on pro-MMP2 by a second molecule of MMP-14, to release activated MMP-2 [47].

Thus, optimal pro-MMP2 activation requires adequate levels of pro-MMP2 and TIMP2 and good mobility of these two components within the matrix of Bruch's to interact with the MMP-14 enzyme on the RPE basal membrane. The age-related reduction in diffusion within Bruch's is expected to compromise this activation potential (**Figure 3**). Furthermore, pro-MMP2 covalently binds pro-MMP9 to form the high molecular weight complex termed HMW2, reducing its level for the activation process [48]. A polymorphism in the microsatellite region of the MMP9 gene (present in most AMD patients) results in elevated levels of pro-MMP9 in both plasma and Bruch's membrane, increasing the potential for further sequestration of pro-MMP2 from the activation step [39, 49–51].

The gross alterations of ageing Bruch's membrane together with the reduction in diffusional competence are expected to hamper the mobility of pro-MMP2 and TIMP2, diminishing the activation of this MMP. Thus, levels of activated MMP2 decrease with age, and in AMD, the level was reduced by 50% compared to age-matched controls [39]. It should also be noted that activated MMP2 may not be able to diffuse adequately to interact with its substrate and in the gross morphology of **Figure 1**, may be trapped within the membrane. The decreased turnover of Bruch's leads to the deleterious morphological and functional changes described earlier culminating in diminished support of RPE and photoreceptors.

2.4.4 Ageing and increased susceptibility to inflammatory intervention

Many of the toxic products produced in the RPE and present in Bruch's (as outlined earlier), including A2E, bis-retinoids, malonaldehyde, carbonyl lipids, C-reactive protein, etc., are capable of activating the complement system [52]. Thus, in elderly subjects, the exponential increase in A2E in Bruch's may be associated with a low-grade complement activation [53, 54]. A low-grade inflammatory response may be beneficial for eliminating toxic metabolites present in Bruch's or in drusen and may serve to prevent the transition from normal ageing to pathology. Thus, the presence of the membrane attack complex and other complement factors in drusen and inter-capillary columns may allow their removal by macrophages [55].

However, indiscriminate activation of the complement system can lead to a chronic inflammatory response damaging RPE and photoreceptor cells. CFH (a 155 kDa glycoprotein) plays important roles in modulating the activation of the complement cascade. Firstly, it can bind to the toxic entities to prevent complement activation and secondly, by binding to the C3b complement component, block the progression of the cascade [56–58].

Levels of CFH in Bruch's are maintained by synthesis in the RPE and binding to glycosaminoglycans in the membrane, and delivery of plasma-derived CFH. With age, and under oxidative stress, the production of CFH by the RPE is reduced [59, 60]. Similarly, the nearly 10-fold decrease in diffusion across elderly Bruch's is expected to compromise delivery from the blood. Furthermore, in the presence of inflammatory activity in Bruch's, CFH is nitrated [61]. This nitrated CFH does not bind lipid peroxidation products nor C3b, diminishing its protective ability. Also, plasma levels of nitrated CFH are elevated in AMD patients and this may contribute to AMD progression [61].

A polymorphism in the CFH gene (Tyr402His) has been detected in about 50% of AMD patients [62, 63]. This mutated CFH shows diminished binding to toxic ligands such as malondialdehyde and C-reactive protein, and thus becomes ineffective in modulating the inflammatory response [64–66]. Mutated CFH also shows poor binding to heparin sulphate in Bruch's and hence its enhanced presence in Bruch's is compromised [67].

Ageing changes in Bruch's and the RPE therefore compromise the protective effects of CFH and in the aged AMD patient may exacerbate the inflammatory response leading to the death of RPE and photoreceptors.

3. Requirements for effective therapeutic intervention in dry AMD

Oxidative damage in the RPE and Bruch's membrane is the primary driver of ageing changes in the normal elderly and more so in patients with AMD. These ageing changes diminish the supply of key anti-oxidants and vitamins required to combat oxidative stress and therefore a vicious cycle is set-up that leads to the degenerative changes in AMD.

Anti-oxidant and vitamin supplement regimes have been devised as a possible interventionist measure to reduce oxidative stress and hopefully slow the progression of the disease. Thus, the AREDS dietary supplementation cocktail was devised (vitamin C (500 mg), vitamin E (400 IU), beta-carotene (15 mg), zinc oxide (80 mg), and cupric oxide (2 mg)) and initial results showed it to be effective in reducing the risk of visual loss [68, 69]. The supplement was further modified (as the AREDS 2 formulation) by removing beta-carotene and adding lutein (10 mg) and zeaxanthine (2 mg) but did not confer any additional benefits [70].

Despite the wide use of AREDS supplements for over 10 years, controversy remains as to its usefulness since it does not prevent legal blindness in advanced AMD [71]. It has been pointed out that the earlier reported decrease in progression was related to the occurrence of neovascularisation rather than slowing the progression of dry AMD [72].

Given the fact that the diffusion of metabolites across Bruch's membrane is reduced by nearly 10-fold in the elderly, and perhaps more so in AMD, one must question the likely effectiveness of such dietary supplementation. The major problem with supplementation therapies is that they do not address transport in the opposite direction across Bruch's membrane i.e., the removal of toxic metabolites that are the likely triggers of neovascular and inflammatory episodes.

For effective therapeutic intervention, it would be ideal to improve the bi-directional transport pathways across Bruch's membrane, to improve nutritional and anti-oxidant delivery and to remove toxic waste products. This would require the destabilisation and dispersal of the lipid-rich debris and the removal of normal and damaged proteinaceous deposits. Such a strategy would also release trapped activated MMP enzymes that could participate in hydrolysing the altered collagenous components. The expected improvement in intra-membrane mobility would favour greater activation of pro-MMP2, kick-starting the normal rejuvenation machinery in Bruch's membrane. Therapeutic success would be realised if the transport decay curves shown in **Figures 2** and **3** could be elevated so that they no longer crossed the failure threshold within the lifetime of an individual. The potential implementation of such a strategy using saponin molecules is discussed next.

4. Saponin characteristics enabling therapeutic intervention in dry AMD

Saponins are amphipathic molecules that have hydrophobic and hydrophilic domains that can partition into lipoidal deposits and assist dispersal [73–76]. Saponins extracted from the ginseng plant (Panax ginseng CA Meyer) have a 4-membered triterpenoid ring and are often referred to as ginsenosides or steroidal glycosides because of the structural similarity to the cholesterol molecule (**Figure 4A**). The type and number of sugar units attached at sites R1, R2, and R3

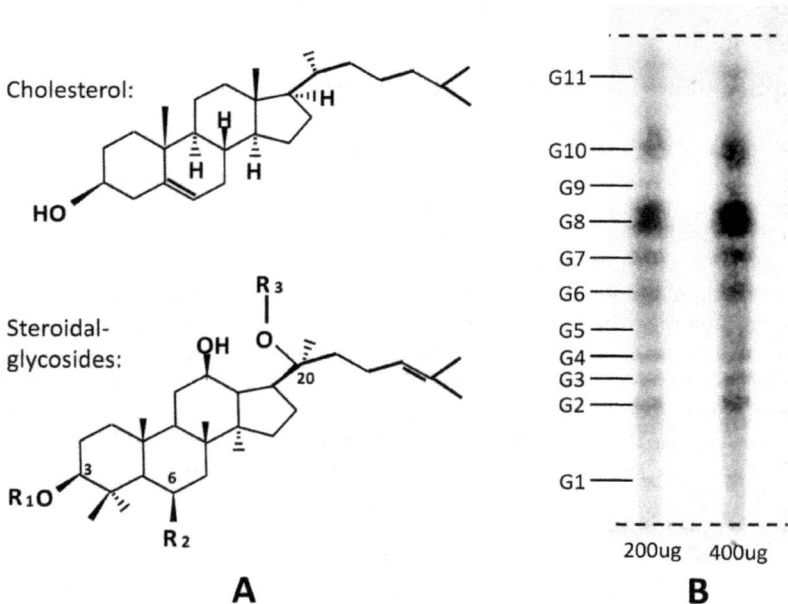

Figure 4.
Saponins extracted from the ginseng plant. (A) Structural similarity of saponins to the cholesterol molecule. Sugar attachment sites R1, R2, and R3 lead to the diversity of saponin species. (B) TLC of extracted saponins. G1 to G11 denote the major spots, each spot comprising several species.

gives rise to a myriad of species and over 30 have been structurally characterised. Saponins extracted from the roots of the ginseng plant were separated on Silica Gel thin-layer-chromatography (TLC) plates using a solvent mixture comprising chloroform: methanol: acetic acid: water (50:30:8:3 v/v) and colour developed by spraying with 20% sulphuric acid in methanol and heating to 100 °C for 5 minutes (**Figure 4B**). Since the separation was dependent on the degree of hydrophilic/hydrophobic properties, each spot on the chromatogram represents a collection of several species.

These saponin molecules not only bind to various lipid classes, they also display transition metal chelating properties [77, 78]. Thus, saponins can chelate the heavy metal deposits in Bruch's membrane and therefore assist in destabilising the lipid aggregates.

4.1 Saponin mediated dispersal of lipid deposits

The potential for saponin mediated dispersal of lipids was assessed in both isolated deposits and intact human Bruch's membrane. Bruch's from four donor eyes (ages 50 and 82 years) was homogenised in Tris-buffer and spun to obtain pellets containing the deposits. Pellets were resuspended in Tris buffer containing ginseng-derived saponins in the range 0-1.2 mg/ml and incubated for 12 hours at 37°C. Samples were then spun and any lipids released into the supernatants extracted with chloroform: methanol (2:1 v/v). Lipids were then separated on Silica Gel thin-layer chromatography (TLC) plates using solvent system #1, chloroform: methanol: acetic acid: water (50:30:8:3 v/v) and solvent system #2, heptane: diethyl ether: acetic acid (70:30:2 v/v). Lipid spots were visualised by staining with amido-black 10B stain and following densitometry, levels quantified with reference to standard curves. Saponins were observed to rapidly release various lipid classes from the deposits in a dose dependent manner (**Figure 5**).

In addition, 14 Bruch's preparations were obtained from 4 human donors (age range 64-75 years) and mounted in Ussing chambers. All chambers were perfused with Tris buffer to remove loosely attached debris and then half the chambers were incubated with Tris buffer and the other half with Tris buffer containing 4.6 mg/ml saponins for 12 hours at 37°C. Chambers were rinsed in Tris buffer and the content of the various lipid classes present in Bruch's membrane quantified as detailed above. The content of lipids in the samples incubated with saponins was significantly reduced compared to controls (**Figure 6**). Thus, saponin molecules are able to solubilise and disperse the lipid deposits in Bruch's membrane.

4.2 Saponin-mediated release of deposited proteins

Soluble proteins that are either damaged due to chemical modification or denatured tend to unfold exposing the hydrophobic regions to the aqueous environment. This leads to aggregation and deposition within Bruch's membrane. The possibility that saponins could interact with these 'amphipathic' structures to de-segregate and solubilise them was also assessed. Bruch's membrane from four human donors (age range 49-77 years) was mounted in 8 Ussing chambers and perfused with Tris buffer. The perfusate was collected every 5 hours and the protein content determined. As indicated in **Figure 7**, perfusion with Tris buffer resulted in slow release of loosely adherent proteins up to the fourth perfusion period (20 hours). In four chambers, the perfusion fluid was then switched to one containing 167 μg/ml of saponin Rb1. This resulted in the rapid and copious release of further, presumably trapped proteins from the membrane (**Figure 7**). The possibility that trapped MMP enzymes may also have been released is assessed below.

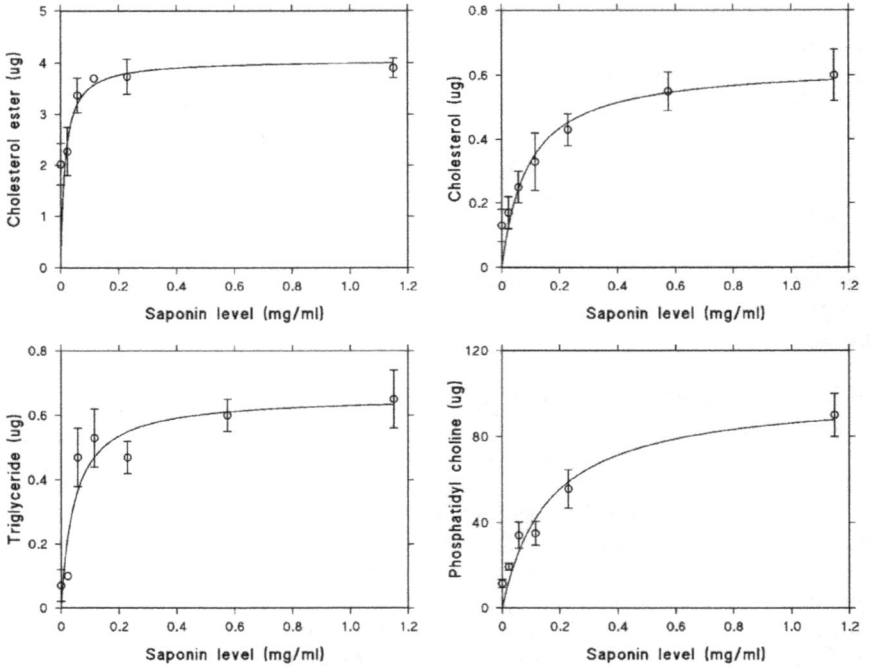

Figure 5.
Saponin-mediated release of lipids from deposits extracted from Bruch's membrane. Extracted deposits were incubated with saponins in the range 0-1.2 mg/ml for 12 hours, spun, and lipids present in the supernatant quantified. Saponins released cholesterol, cholesterol esters, phospholipids, and triglycerides in a dose-dependent manner. Data is given as Mean ± SD.

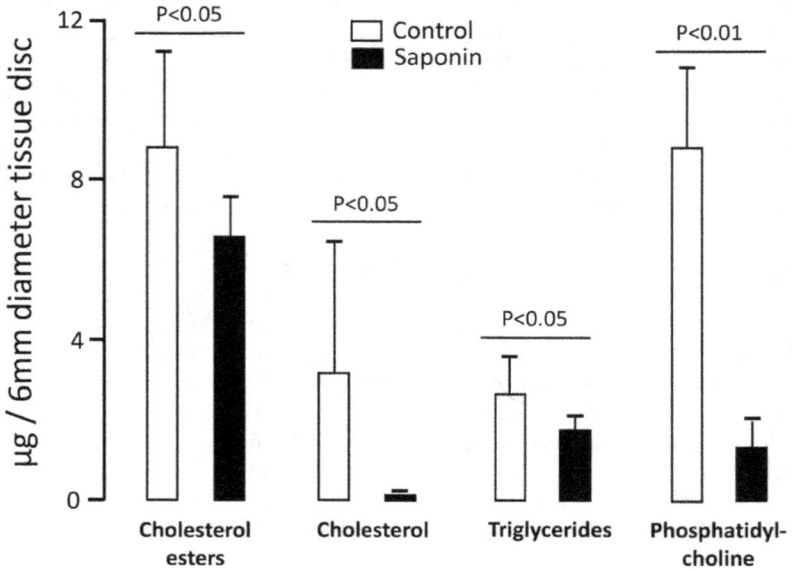

Figure 6.
Saponin-mediated release of lipids from intact human Bruch's membrane. The level of the major lipid classes was reduced following saponin treatment. Data is given as Mean ± SD.

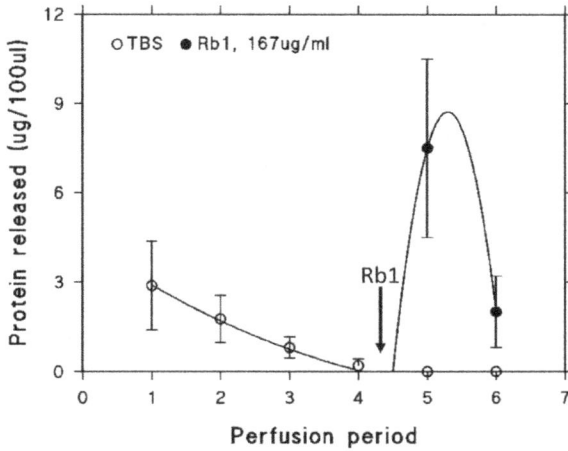

Figure 7.
Solubilisation and release of trapped proteins from Bruch's membrane. On perfusion with saline, loosely adherent proteins are released slowly. When there was no further release (after period 4), the perfusion medium was switched to one containing Rb1, resulting in the copious release of trapped proteins. TBS-Tris buffered saline; Rb1-Ginsenoside Rb1. Data as Mean ± SD.

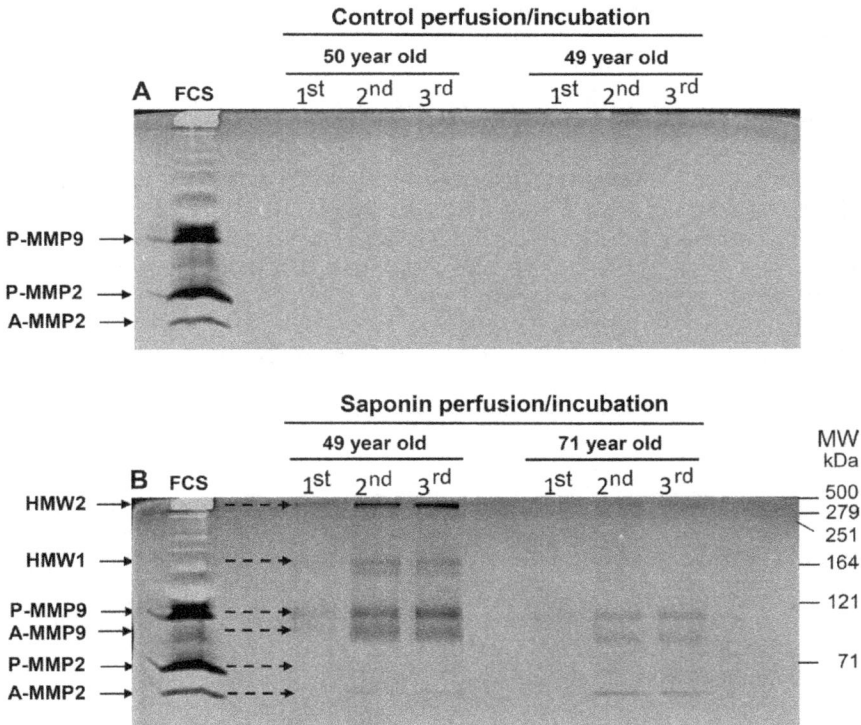

Figure 8.
Saponin-mediated release of trapped MMP enzymes. (A) Perfusion with Tris buffer did not release any MMP species from Bruch's membrane. (B) Saponin perfusion released trapped MMP species and in particular activated forms of MMPs 2&9. FCS-foetal calf serum standard. P- pro-MMPs; A-activated MMPs. From reference [43].

4.3 Saponin-mediated release of trapped MMP enzymes

MMPs are detected by the technique of gelatine zymography. This is standard electrophoresis but with the gel containing 1% gelatine, a substrate for MMPs. Samples are electrophoresed with the MMPs migrating according to molecular weight, the smaller ones running fastest. Following electrophoresis, the gel is incubated in Tris-buffer (containing calcium) for a period of 18-24 hours to allow the MMP enzymes to digest the gelatine in their locality. The gel is then stained with Coomassie Blue and after de-staining, regions containing gelatine stain blue but where the gelatine has been hydrolysed (by MMP enzymes), the region is colourless. Reversing the grey-scale of the gel image shows the MMP regions as dark bands and the identity of the MMP is confirmed from its molecular weight.

To assess the likely effect of saponins on release of trapped MMP enzymes, Bruch's membrane from donors aged 49-71 years was mounted in Ussing chambers and perfused for a period of 12 hours to remove plasma-derived and loosely bound MMP species. Half the chambers were then perfused with Tris buffer for three periods of 3 hours each and the remaining half with saponins at a level of 4.6 mg/ml. After each period, the perfusate was collected and examined by zymography. Incubation with Tris did not show the release of any MMP species (**Figure 8A**). However, perfusion with saponins showed a trace release of MMPs in the first period followed by greater release in the two subsequent periods (**Figure 8B**). The release profiles showed the presence of activated MMP9 and MMP2. If this release occurred in vivo, it would kick start the MMP degradation machinery, rejuvenating the membrane.

5. Functional improvement of Bruch's membrane

Saponins have been shown to disperse and release lipid deposits, protein aggregates and trapped active MMP enzymes as described earlier. This is akin to reversing the ageing process of Bruch's membrane. The likely impact of these changes on the functional properties of Bruch's has also been assessed by monitoring hydraulic conductivity and diffusional status.

5.1 Hydraulic conductivity of saponin treated human Bruch's

Hydraulic conductivity measurements were undertaken in 23 preparations of Bruch's membrane from donors over the age range 13-90 years. After determining basal hydraulic conductivity, samples were incubated with saponins (4.6 mg/ml) for 24 hours at 37°C. After a thorough rinse in Tris buffer, the hydraulic conductivity was re-assessed. Treatment with saponins improved the hydraulic conductivity about 2-fold (p < 0.0001) elevating the exponential decay curves upwards, away from the failure threshold (**Figure 9**).

The curves were shifted by 19 years, reversing the ageing decline in fluid transport. Such a shift means that the curves will meet the failure threshold outside the normal human life span. In AMD, this improvement will reduce the risk of pigment epithelial detachments that normally affects 12-20% of these patients. These results were obtained after a single exposure to the saponins. A second subsequent exposure to the saponins (1.15 mg/ml) further increased the improvement in hydraulic conductivity indicative of potential to further elevate the decay curves (**Figure 10**). This is the likely result of continued removal of lipid and protein debris and release of MMP enzymes.

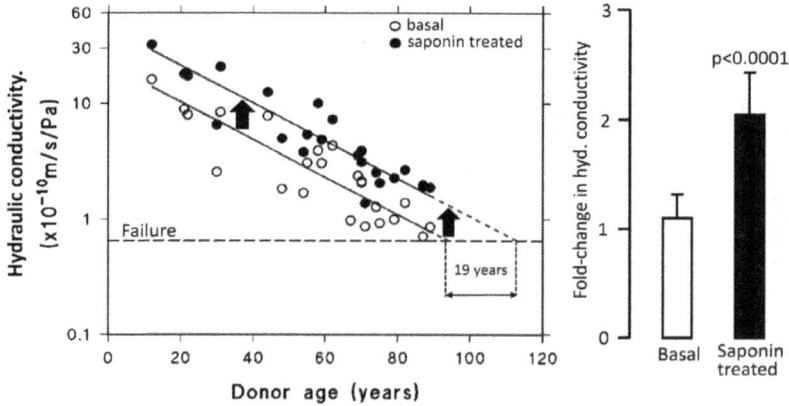

Figure 9.
Effect of saponins on the hydraulic conductivity of human Bruch's membrane. Saponins improved the hydraulic conductivity by 2-fold across the age range examined (p<0.0001). Decay curves were elevated so that failure threshold was met 19 years later. Modified from reference [43].

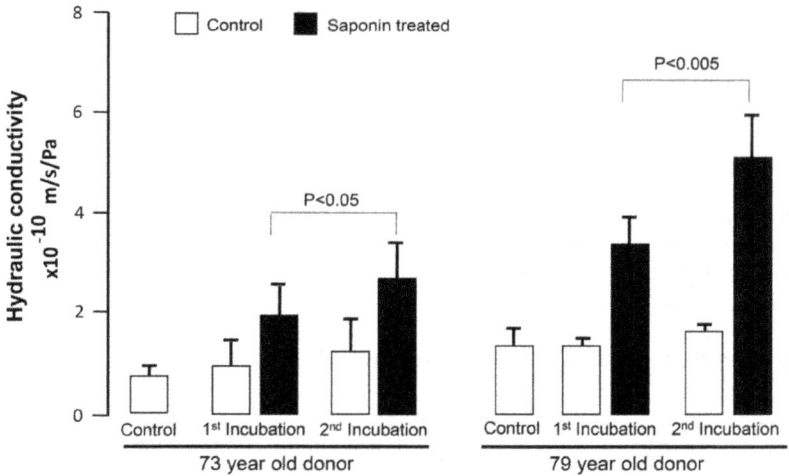

Figure 10.
Effect of repeated saponin exposure on the hydraulic conductivity of Bruch's membrane. Initial exposure to saponins improved hydraulic conductivity by over 2-fold. This was further increased by a second exposure.

5.2 Diffusional status of saponin treated human Bruch's

Diffusional status of Bruch's was assessed by following the transport of an FITC-labelled albumin test molecule (MW 65 kDa, hydrodynamic radius 3.5 nm) across the membrane, at a concentration gradient of 0.1 mM. Bruch's was obtained from 21 human donors (age range 12-92 years) and the basal diffusion rate was first determined. After a thorough wash in Tris buffer for 3 hours to remove all traces of albumin, the samples were incubated with saponin solution (4.6 mg/ml) for 24 hours at 37°C. Following a rinse with Tris buffer, the diffusional status was re-assessed. Exposure to saponins improved the diffusional status of Bruch's membrane by 2-fold (p<0.0001) shifting the ageing decay lines upwards, effectively reversing the ageing process by ~15 years (**Figure 11**).

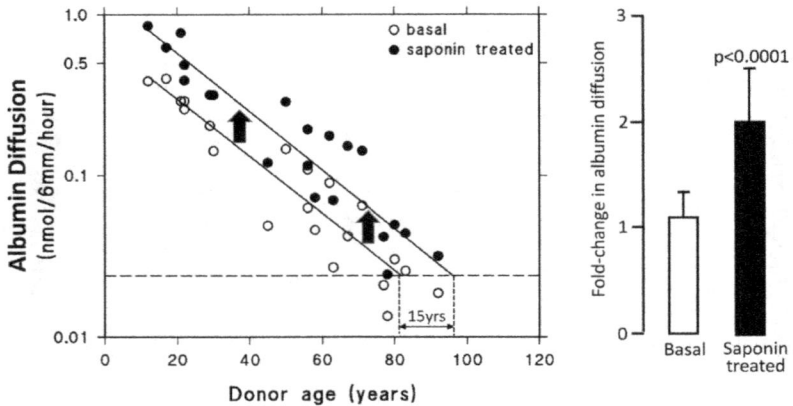

Figure 11.
Effect of saponins on the diffusional status of Bruch's membrane. Saponin incubation improved diffusion (p<0.0001) elevating the decay curves upwards so that they reached failure thresholds 15 years later. Modified from reference [43].

Saponin mediated improvement in diffusion within Bruch's membrane would allow greater delivery of nutrients, vitamins and anti-oxidants to both the RPE and photoreceptor cells. Reduction in oxidative stress would result in reduced production of A2E and other bis-retinoids minimising the generation of pro-inflammatory mediators. Similarly, the removal of toxic waste products from Bruch's would be facilitated. This would also improve the mobility of TIMP2 and proMMP2 allowing greater activation of the MMP species and thus improved turnover of Bruch's membrane. Furthermore, improved mobility of CFH would minimise the risk of inflammatory involvement. In AMD, these changes are expected to slow the degenerative phase of the disease.

6. Conclusions: potential for saponin-mediated therapy in dry AMD

In-vitro work, using donor human Bruch's preparations has demonstrated the potential for saponin molecules to disperse and remove lipoidal and proteinaceous debris, releasing trapped activated MMP enzymes that can then mediate the normal degradation processes essential for rejuvenation of the membrane. Associated with these changes was a significant improvement in the bi-directional transport properties of Bruch's membrane. In vivo, improved transport would considerably augment the delivery of protective anti-oxidants and related nutrients to the RPE and photoreceptor cells and more importantly stimulate the removal of toxic products that underlie the progression of the disease.

Saponins constitute a large mixture of amphipathic molecules, the diversity being due to the varied nature of sugar residues at the several attachment sites on the aglycone ring structure. Individual species, such as ginsenoside Rb1 or Compound K have been shown to improve the functional status of Bruch's membrane preparations [43]. These compounds could be administered by intra-ocular injection as a potential therapy. But being very difficult to synthesise, reliance would have to be on isolation and purification from natural sources and therefore not likely to be cost-effective.

The alternative would be to utilise a varied mixture of saponins and this has many advantages. Firstly, they can be administered orally and in the Far East have been used as nutritional supplements for centuries. Secondly, and most importantly, a mixture can target a broad spectrum of substrates that are normally encountered in the deposits in Bruch's membrane. From the pharmacokinetic data currently available for saponins, and our in-vitro dose response curves, calculations suggest that a 200 mg dose of an appropriate saponin mixture, taken twice daily, should significantly improve the transport characteristics of Bruch's membrane over a period of 4-6 months. Work is in progress to develop a clinical protocol for assessing the usefulness of saponin-mediated therapy for dry AMD.

Unlike other therapeutic interventions in AMD where outcome has been judged by following the progression of the disease over a period of 2-5 years, the saponin intervention can be assessed at 4-6 months using dark-adaptation kinetics. Since the saponin intervention aims at improving the transport systems in Bruch's membrane, the increased delivery of vitamin A would supplement the retinoid stores in the RPE allowing faster delivery of 11-cis retinal to the photoreceptor, and hence faster dark adaptation would be expected as proof of principle of saponin intervention.

Author details

Yunhee Lee[1], Eun Jung Ahn[2] and Ali Hussain[3*]

1 AltRegen Co., Ltd. 12 Bongeunsa-ro 47-gil, Seoul, Republic of Korea

2 Daehakro Seoul Eye Clinic, Seoul, Republic of Korea

3 Department of Ocular Biology and Therapeutics, UCL Institute of Ophthalmology, London, UK

*Address all correspondence to: alyhussain@aol.com

IntechOpen

References

[1] Li JQ, Welchowski T, Schmid M, Mauschitz MM, Holz FG, Finger RP. Prevalence and incidence of age-related macular degeneration in Europe: a systematic review and meta-analysis. Br. J. Ophthalmol. 2020; 104:1077-1084.

[2] Bressler NM. Antiangiogenic approaches to age-related macular degeneration today. Ophthalmology, 2009;116(10. Suppl.):15-23.

[3] Ba J, Peng R-S, Xu D, Li Y-H, Shi H, Wang Q, Yu J. Intravitreal anti-VEGF injections for treating wet age-related macular degeneration: a systematic review and meta-analysis. Drug Design, Development and Therapy 2015; 9:5397-5405.

[4] Van Newkirk MR, Nanjan MB, Wang JJ, Mitchell P, Taylor HR, McCarthy CA. The prevalence of age-related maculopathy: the visual impairment project. Ophthalmol. 2000; 107:1593-1600.

[5] Majewski J, Schultz DW, Weleber RG, Schain MB, Edwards AO, Matise TC, et al. Age-related macular degeneration – a genome scan in extended families. Am. J. Hum. Genet. 2003; 73:540-550.

[6] Seddon JM, Santangelo SL, Book K, Chong S, Cote J. A genome wide scan for age-related macular degeneration provides for linkage to several chromosomal regions. Am. J. Hum. Genet. 2003; 73:780-790.

[7] Murdaugh LS, Wang Z, Del Priore LV, Dillon J, Gaillard ER. Age-related accumulation of 3-nitrotyrosine and nitro-A2E in human Bruch's membrane. Exp. Eye Res. 2010; 90:564-571.

[8] Liu J, Itagaki Y, Ben-Shabat S, Nakanishi K, Sparrow JR. The biosynthesis of A2E, a fluophore of ageing retina, involves the formation of the precursor, A2-PE, in the photoreceptor outer membrane. J. Biol. Chem. 2000; 275, 29354-29360.

[9] Sparrow JR, Gregory-Roberts E, Yamamoto K, Blonska A, Ghosh SK, Ueda K, Zhou J. The bisretinoids of retinal pigment epithelium Prog. Ret. Res. 2012; 31: 121-135.

[10] Wu Y, Yanase E, Feng X, Siegel MM, Sparrow JR (2010) Structural characterization of bisretinoid A2E photocleavage products and implications for age-related macular degeneration. Proc. Natl. Acad. Sci. 2010; 107: 7275-7280.

[11] Liu A, Chang J, Lin Y, Shen Z, Bernstein PS. Long-chain and very long chain polyunsaturated fatty acids in ocular ageing and age-related macular degeneration. J. Lipid Res. 2010; 51:3217-3229.

[12] Lu L, Gu X, Hong X, Laird J, Jaffe K, Choi J, Crabb JW, Salomon RG. Synthesis and structural characterization of carboxyethylpyrrole-modified proteins: mediators of age-related macular degeneration. Biorg. Med. Chem. 2009; 17:7548-7561.

[13] Gu X, Meer SG, Miyagi M, Rayborn ME, Hollyfield JG, Crabb JW, Salomon RG: Carboxyethylpyrrole protein adducts and autoantibodies, biomarkers for age-related macular degeneration. J. Biol. Chem. 2003, 278:42027-42035.

[14] Oliver PD, Newsome DA. Mitochondrial superoxide dismutase in mature and developing human retinal pigment epithelium. Invest. Ophthalmol. Vis. Sci. 1992; 33:1909-1918.

[15] Sternberg P, Davidson PC, Jones DP, Hagen TM, Reed RL, Drews-Botsch C. Protection of retinal pigment epithelium from oxidative injury by glutathione and precursors. Invest. Ophthalmol. Vis. Sci. 1993; 34:3661-3668.

[16] Ng KP, Gugiu B, Renganathan K, Davies MW, Gu X, Crabb JS, Kim SR, Rozanowska MB, Bonilha VL, Rayborn ME, Salomon RG, Sparrow JR, Boulton ME, Hollyfield JG, Crabb JW. Retinal pigment epithelium Lipofuscin proteomics. Mol. Cell Proteomics 2008; 7:1397-1405.

[17] Bergmann M, Scutt F, Holz FG, Kopitz J. Inhibition of the ATP-driven proton pump in RPE lysosomes by the major lipofuscin fluorophore A2E may contribute to the pathogenesis of age-related macular degeneration. FASEB J. 2004; 18(3):562-564.

[18] Feeney-Burns L, Hilderbrand ES, Eldridge S. Aginghuman RPE – morphometric analysis of macular, equatorial, and peripheral cells. Invest Ophthalmol Vis Sci 1984; 25:195-200.

[19] Uchiki T., Weikel KA., Jiao W., et al., (2012) Glycation-altered proteolysis as a pathobiologic mechanism that links glycemic index, aging, and age-related macular disease. Aging Cell 2012; 11(1): 1-13.

[20] Inana G, Murat C, An W, Yao X, Harris I, Cao J. RPE phagocytic function declines in age-related macular degeneration and is rescued by human umbilical tissue derived cells. J. Transl. Med. 2018; 16:63.

[21] Barron MJ, Johnson MA, Andrews RM, Clarke MP, Griffiths PG, Bristow E, He L-P, Durham S, Turnbul DM. Mitochondrial abnormalities in ageing macular photoreceptors. Invest. Ophthalmol. Vis. Sci. 2001; 42:3016-3022.

[22] Suter M, Reme C, Grimm C et al. Age-related macular degeneration: The lipofuscin component retinyl-n-retinylidene ethanolamine detaches proapoptotic proteins from mitochondria and induces apoptosis in mammalian retinal pigment epithelial cells. J. Biol. Chem. 2000; 275:39625-39630.

[23] Wielgus A, Collier R, Martin E, et al. Blue light induced A2E oxidation in rat eyes-experimental animal model of dry AMD. Photochem. Photobiol. Sci. 2010; 9:1505-1512.

[24] Jackson GR, Owsley C, McGwin G. Aging and dark adaptation. Vis. Res. 1999; 38, 3655-3662.

[25] Owsley C, Jackson GR, White M, Feist R, Edwards DJ. Delays in rod-mediated dark adaptation in early age-related maculopathy. Ophthalmology. 2001; 108: 1196-1202.

[26] Owsley C, McGwin G, Jackson GR, Heinburger DC, Piyathilake CJ, Klein R, White MF, Kallies K. Effect of short term, high-dose retinol on dark adaptation in age and age-related maculopathy. Invest. Ophthalmol. Vis. Sci. 2006; 47(4): 1310-1318.

[27] Quinn RH & Miller SS. Ion transport mechanisms in native human retinal pigment epithelium. Invest. Ophthalmol. Vis. Sci. 1992; 33: 3513-3527.

[28] Bialek S & Miller SS. K+ and Cl- transport mechanisms in bovine pigment epithelium that could modulate subretinal space, volume and composition. J. Physiol. 1994; 475: 401-417.

[29] Chihara E and Nao-I N. Resorption of subretinal fluid by transepithelial flow of the retinal pigment epithelium. Graefes Arch. Klin. Exp. Ophthalmol. 1985; 223: 202-204.

[30] Tsuboi S. Measurement of the volume flow and hydraulic conductivity across the isolated dog retinal pigment epithelium. Invest. Ophthalmol. Vis. Sci. 1987; 28: 21776-21782.

[31] Okubo A, Rosa RH, Bunce CV, Alexander RA, Fan JT, Bird AC and Luthert PJ. The relationships of age changes in retinal pigment epithelium and Bruch's membrane. Invest. Ophthalmol. Vis. Sci. 1999; 40: 443-449.

[32] Karwatowski WSS, Jefferies TE, Duance VC, Albon J, Bailey AJ & Easty DL. Preparation of Bruch's membrane and analysis of the age-related changes in the structural collagens. Brit. J. Ophthalmol. 1995; 79: 944-952.

[33] Handa JT, Verzijl N, Matsunaga H, Aotaki-Keen A, Lutty GA, te Koppele JM, Miyata T and Hjelmeland LM. Increase in the advanced glycation end-product pentosidine in Bruch's membrane with age. Invest. Ophthalmol. Vis. Sci. 1999; 40: 775-779.

[34] Holz FG, Sheraidah GS, Pauleikhoff D and Bird AC. Analysis of lipid deposits extracted from human macular and peripheral Bruch's membrane. Arch. Ophthalmol. 1994; 112: 402-406.

[35] Ruberti JW, Curcio CA, Millican CL, Menco BPM, Huang JD, Johnson M. Quick freeze/deep-etch visualization of age-related lipid accumulation in Bruch's membrane. Invest. Ophthalmol. Vis. Sci. 2003; 44:1753-1759.

[36] Anderson DH., MullinsRF., Hageman GS., Johnson LV. A role for local inflammation in the formation of drusen in the aging eye. Am J Ophthalmol. 2012; 34(3), 411-431.

[37] Lengyl I, Finn TM, Pelo T et al. High concentration of zinc in sub-retinal pigment epithelial deposits. Exp. Eye Res. 2007; 84:727-780.

[38] Hussain AA, Lee Y, Marshall J. Understanding the complexity of the matrix metalloproteinase system and its relevance to age-related diseases: Age-related macular degeneration and Alzheimer's disease. Prog. Ret. Eye Res. 2020; 74:100775.

[39] Hussain AA, Lee Y, Zhang JJ, Marshall J. Disturbed matrix metalloproteinase activity of Bruch's membrane in age-related macular degeneration. Invest. Ophthalmol. Vis. Sci. 2011; 52:4459-4466.

[40] Hussain AA., Starita C., and Marshall J. (2004) Chapter IV. Transport characteristics of ageing human Bruch's membrane: Implications for AMD. In: Focus on Macular Degeneration Research, (Editor O. R. Ioseliani). 2004. p. 59-113. Nova Science Publishers, Inc. New York.

[41] Curcio CA, Johnson M. Structure, function, and pathology of Bruch's membrane. In: Ryan SJ, ed. Retina. St. Louis, MO: Mosby-Year Book. 2013. p.465-481.

[42] Bird AC & Marshall J. Retinal pigment epithelial detachments in the elderly. Trans. Soc. Ophthal. UK. 1986; 105: 674-682.

[43] Lee Y, Hussain AA, Seok J-H, Kim S-H, Marshall J. Modulating the transport characteristics of Bruch's membrane with steroidal glycosides and its relevance to age-related macular degeneration (AMD). Invest. Ophthalmol. Vis. Sci. 2015; 56:8403-8418.

[44] Moore DJ and Clover GM. The effect of age on the macromolecular permeability of human Bruch's membrane. Invest. Ophthalmol. Vis. Sci. 2001; 42: 2970-2975.

[45] Hussain AA, Starita C, Hodgetts A, Marshall J. Macromolecular diffusion characteristics of ageing human Bruch's

membrane: implications for age-related macular degeneration (AMD). Exp. Eye Res. 2010; 90:703-710.

[46] Woessner JF. Matrix metalloproteinases and their inhibitors in connective tissue remodelling. FASEB J. 1991; 5:2145-2154.

[47] Butler, GS., Butler, MJ., Atkinson, SJ., Will, H., Tamura, T., Schade van Westrum, S., Crabbe, T., Clements J., d'Ortho, MP. and Murphy, G. The TIMP-2 membrane type I metalloproteinase 'receptor' regulates the concentration and efficient activation of progelatinase A: a kinetic study. J Biol. Chem. 1998; 273:871-880.

[48] Kumar A, El-Osta A, Hussain AA, Marshall J. Increased sequestration of matrix metalloproteinases in ageing human Bruch's membrane: Implications for ECM turnover. Invest. Ophthalmol. Vis. Sci. 2010; 51:2664-2670.

[49] Fornoni A, Wang Y, Lenz O, Dtriker LJ, Striker GE. Association of a decreased number of d(CA) repeats in the matrix metalloproteinase-9 promoter with glomerulosclerosis susceptibility in mice. J. Am. Soc. Nephrol. 2002; 13:2068-2076.

[50] Fiotti N, Pedio M, Battaglia PM, Atamura N, Uxa L, et al. MMP-9 microsatellite polymorphism and susceptibility to exudative form of age-related macular degeneration. Genet. Med. 2007; 4:272-277.

[51] Chau KY, Sivaprasad S, Patel N, Donaldson TA, Luthert PJ, Chong NV. Plasma levels of matrix metalloproteinase-2 and –9 (MMP2 and MMP9) in age-related macular degeneration. Eye (Lond.) 2008; 22:855-859.

[52] Jang YP, Matsuda H, Itagaki Y, Nakanishi K, Sparrow JR: Characterization of peroxy-A2E and furan-A2E photo-oxidation products and detection in human and mouse retinal pigment epithelium cell Lipofuscin. J. Biol. Chem. 2005; 280:39732-39739.

[53] Anderson DH, Radeke MJ, Gallo NB, Chapin EA, Johnson PT, Curletti CR, Hancox LS, et al.: The pivotal role of the complement system in ageing and age-related macular degeneration: hypothesis re-visited. Prog Retin Eye Res. 2010; 29:95-112.

[54] Khandhadia S, Cipriani V, Yates JRW, Lottery AJ: Age-related macular degeneration and the complement system. Immunobiology, 2012; 217:127-146.

[55] Crabb JW, Miyagi M, Gu X, Shadrach K, West KA, Sakaguchi H, Kamei M, Hasan A, YanI, Rayborn ME, Salomon RG, Hollyfield JG. Drusen proteome analysis: an approach to the aetiology of age-related macular degeneration. Proc. Natl. Acad. Sci. USA. 2002; 99, 14682-14687.

[56] De Cordoba SR, Esparza-Gordillo J, de Jorge DE, Lopez-Trascasa M, Sanchez-Corral P. The human complement factor H: functional roles, genetic variations and disease associations. Mol. Immunol. 2004; 41:355-367.

[57] Makou E, Herbert AP, Barlow PN. Functional anatomy of complement factor H. Biochem. 2013; 52:3949-3962.

[58] Weismann D, Hartvigsen K, Lauer N, BennettKL, Scholl HP, Charbel Issa P, Cano M, Brandstatter H, Tsimikas S, Skerka C, Superti-Furga G, Handa JT, Zipfel PF, Witzum JL, Binder CJ. Complement factor H binds lamondialdehyde epitopes and protects from oxidative stress. Nature, 2011; 478:76-81.

[59] Bian Q, Gao S, Zhou J, Qin J, Taylor A, Hohnson EJ, Tang G, Sparrow JR, Gierhart D, Shang F. Lutein

and zeaxanthine supplementation reduces photo-oxidative damage and modulates the expression of inflammation-related genes in retinal pigment epithelial cells. Free Radic. Biol. Med. 2012; 53:1298-1307.

[60] Lau LI, Chiou SH, Liu CJ, Yen MY, Wei YH. The effect of photo-oxidative stress and inflammatory cytokine on complement factor H expression in retinal pigment epithelial cells. Invest. Ophthalmol. Vis. Sci. 2011; 52:6832-6841.

[61] Krilis M, Qi M, Madigan MC, Wong JWH, et al. Nitration of tyrosines in complement factor H domains alters its immunological activity and mediates a pathogenic role in age-related macular degeneration. Oncotarget. 2017; 8:49016-49032.

[62] Hageman GS, Anderson DH, Johnson LV, Hancox LS, Taiber AJ, Hardisty LI, et al. A common haplotype in the complement regulatory gene factor H (HFI/CFH) predisposes individuals to age-related macular degeneration. Proc. Nat. Acad. Sci USA. 2005; 102:7227-7232

[63] Edwards AO, Ritter R III, Abel KJ, Manning A, Panhuysen C, Farrer LA. Complement factor H polymorphism and age-related macular degeneration. Science 2005; 308:421-424.

[64] Sjoberg AP, Trouw LA, Clark SJ, Sjolander J, Heinegard D, Sim RB, Day AJ, Blom AM. The factor H variant associated with age-related macular degeneration (His-384) and the non-disease-associated form bind differtiually to C-reactive protein, fibromodulin, DNA, and necrotic cells. J. Biol. Chem. 2007; 282:10894-10900.

[65] Lauer N, Mihlan M, Hartmann A, Schlotzer-Schrehardt U, Keilhauer C, Scholl HP, Charbel Issa P, Holz F, Weber BH, Skerka C, Zipfel PF.

Complement regulation at necrotic cell lesions is impaired by the age-related macular degeneration-associated factor-H His402 risk variant. J. Immunol. 2011; 187:4374-4383.

[66] Ferreira VP, Pangburn MK, Cortes C. Complement control protein factor H: the good, the bad, and the inadequate. Mol. Immunol. 2010; 47:2187-2197.

[67] Clark SJ, Perveen R, Hakobyan S, Morganb BP, Sim RB, Bishop PN, Day AJ. (2010). Impaired binding of the age-related macular degeneration-associated complement factor H 402H allotype to Bruch's membrane in human retina. J Biol. Chem. 2010; 285:30192-30202.

[68] Age-Related Eye Disease Study Research Group. A randomized, placebo controlled, clinical trial of high-dose supplementation with vitamins C and E, beta carotene, and zinc for age-related macular degeneration and vision loss: AREDS report no. 8. Arch. Ophthalmol. 2001; 119:1417-1436.

[69] Chew EY, Clemons TE, Agron E, Sperduto RD, SanGiovanni JP, Kurinij N, Davis MD, 2013. Long-term effects of vitamins C and E, beta-carotene, and zinc on age-related macular degeneration. AREDS report No. 35. Ophthalmology. 2013; 120(8):1604-1611.

[70] Age-Related Eye Study 2 (AREDS2) Research Group. Lutein + zeaxanthine and omega-3 fatty acids for age-related macular degeneration: the age-related eye disease study 2 (AREDS2) randomized clinical trial. JAMA. 2013; 309:2005-2015.

[71] Evans JR and Lawrenson JG. Antioxidant vitamin and mineral supplements for preventing age-related macular degeneration. Cochrane Database Syst. Rev. 2017. Jul 30; 7(7):CD000253.

[72] Desmettre T. Geographic atrophy and micronutritional supplements: A complex relationship. J. Fr. Ophthalmol. 2019; 42(10):1111-1115.

[73] Yu BS, Kim A, Chung HH, Yoshikawa W, Akutsu H, Kyogoku Y. Effects of purified ginseng saponins on multilamellar liposomes. Chem. Biol. Interactions. 1985; 56:303-319.

[74] Lee SJ, Lee MH, Lee K. Surface activities of ginseng saponins and their interactions with biomolecules, I. Separations and surface activities of major saponins from fresh ginseng roots. Korean Biochem. J. 1985; 14:1.

[75] Qiu J, Li W, Feng SH, Wang M, He ZY. Ginsenoside Rh2 promotes nonamyloidgenic cleavage of amyloid precursor protein via a cholesterol-dependent pathway. Genet. Mol. Res. 2014; 13: 3586-3598.

[76] Yun U-J, Lee J-H, Koo KH, et al. Lipid raft modulation by Rp1 reverses multidrug resistance via inactivating MDR-1 and Src inhibition. Biochem. Pharmacol. 2013; 85:1441-1453.

[77] Kang KS, Yokozawa T, Yamabe N, Kim HY, Park JH. ESR study on the structure and hydroxyl radical-scavenging activity relationships of ginsenosides isolated from Panax ginseng C.A. Meyer. Biol. Pharm. Bull. 2007; 30:917-921.

[78] Kitts DD, Wijewickreme AN, Hu C. Antioxidant properties of a North American ginseng extract. Mol. Cell Biochem. 2000; 203:1-10.

Section 4

Vision Rehabilitation

Chapter 7

Low-Vision Rehabilitation with Audio-Biofeedback in Age-Related Macular Degeneration

Giovanni Sato and Roberta Rizzo

Abstract

Audio-biofeedback (AFBF) with microperimetry is an important step in low-vision rehabilitation in age-related macular degeneration (AMD). After identifying the preferential retinal locus (PRL) with microperimetry, it is possible to begin rehabilitation to stabilize the PRL, increasing the quality of vision with 10 sessions of audio-biofeedback, at least one session per week, of 10 minutes for each eye. This involves presenting a chessboard grid in the site of fixation variable from the beginning to the end of the session. Audio-biofeedback allows for shifting the site of fixation to another point if the spontaneous fixation that the patient has found is not good to continue rehabilitation; at the end of biofeedback, we call this site the trained retinal locus (TRL) to differentiate it from the PRL. With audio-biofeedback, the low-vision patient with AMD acquires awareness about the best site of vision, thus improving the quality of vision, including better contrast sensitivity, visual acuity, color perception, and definition of the surrounding world.

Keywords: maculopathy, low vision, rehabilitation, preferential retinal locus (PRL), audio-biofeedback (ABFB), microperimetry (MP), bivariate contour ellipse area (BCEA), trained retinal locus (TRL), best corrected visual acuity (BCVA)

1. Introduction

Age-related macular degeneration (AMD) is the primary cause of low vision in the Western world. Patients with low vision typically request treatment so that they can read, write, perform work, recognize faces, watch TV, drive a car, and so on. The damage induced by AMD leads to a central absolute or relative scotoma of different shape and extension, with subsequent loss or reduction of fine visual abilities like reading. Visual rehabilitation in AMD must begin with highlighting the vision needs of the patient. In most cases, being able to read is the first requirement. Face recognition is also very important, particularly when the visually impaired person is greeted by someone they cannot recognize, which may cause embarrassment and potential depression. The recovery of vision in intermediate visual activities such as writing, using the computer, and fine manual work are also fundamental, as is vision for watching television and movies.

The first step in visual rehabilitation is evaluating the patient's residual vision for far and near, which can be unilateral or bilateral. This must be followed by determining the preferential retinal locus (PRL), which can be located above the macula atrophy, nasally, temporally, or inferiorly. The choice of mono or binocular optical aids for reading and distance vision is linked to the location of the PRL and the extent of the scotoma and the residual retina. It is essential to perform a series of orthoptic training for the localization and development of eccentric fixation, until the visually impaired patient becomes aware of their recovery abilities, being able to direct their gaze to the healthy retinal locus corresponding to the PRL. It is a long path that varies according to the depth of the low vision and the depth of the scotoma.

2. Audio-biofeedback

Audio-biofeedback (ABFB) is a process through which the subject learns and regains the ability to control and influence their own physiological responses through one psycho-physiological feedback and greater proprioception [1]. Bio-feedback is used in rehabilitation and is based on biomechanical and physiological measurements of the body such as the neuromuscular, respiratory, and cardiovas-cular systems, movements, postural control, and force. An example of physiological biofeedback is electromyography biofeedback to increase the activity in weak or paretic muscles or to reduce the tone in spastic muscles. In electromyography, surface electrodes are used to detect a change in skeletal muscle activity, which is then fed back to the user by a visual or auditory signal. Another example is cardio-vascular biofeedback, which is used to reduce blood pressure in hypertension and lower the mean heart rate [2].

In ophthalmology, audio-biofeedback is used in low-vision rehabilitation of maculopathy [3]. In our study, patients received eight monocular training sessions of audio-biofeedback, each lasting 10 minutes, every 7 days. Microperimetry (MP-1, Nidek Tech., Padova, Italy) was performed at the beginning and at the end of the sequence, as well as ETDRS visual acuity (VA) at 4 meters and Pelli-Robson Contrast Sensitivity (CS) at 1 meter.

Audio-biofeedback employs a sound to train the patient to keep a specific gaze position, which is marked on the digital retinal image by the operator and displayed as a target to the patient. If the patient's gaze matches the selected position, a continuous sound is emitted. When the eye drifts away, the sound becomes pro-gressively more discontinuous.

The contribution of audio-biofeedback to low-vision rehabilitation depends on the seriousness of the case, although it is useful in all cases. In some cases, where the PRL is in a good place, biofeedback allows stabilization of a fixation already used with the increase of retinal sensitivity in decibel and reduction of the fixation ellipse known as the bivariate contour ellipse area (BCEA).

In other cases, where the PRL used by the patient is in an area of little use for vision with an insufficient visual span to reading, audio-biofeedback allows shifting of the fixation to a better locus called the trained retinal locus (TRL).

2.1 Features and parameters of audio biofeedback

In audio-biofeedback with microperimetry, tracking is one of the key features, as it allows for automatic detecting of the patient's eye movements during the exam of fixation as well as during the feedback training. The tracking detects and scores the patient's fixation trajectory frame by frame. The user can preconfigure the parameters that define the characteristics of the fixation target, including the shape, extent, color, and thickness of the target.

There is the possibility to use letters or phrases as "custom" fixation.

The stability of fixation is classified [4–6] as follows:

1. Stable if more than 75% of the fixation points are contained within the circle with a diameter equal to 2°.

2. Relatively unstable if more than 75% of the fixation points are contained within the circle with a diameter of 2°.

3. Unstable if less than 75% of the fixation points are contained within the circle with a diameter of 4°.

The fixation itself is classified as follows:

a. Predominant central if more than 50% of the fixation points are contained within the foveal circle with a diameter of 2°.

b. Poorly central if the fixation points contained within the foveal circle are between 25% and 50%.

c. Predominantly eccentric if less than 25% of the fixation points are contained within the circle fixation trajectory.

The area of fixation is called bivariate contour ellipse area (BCEA) and is based on the published scientific literature [7]. The results of the relative analysis are converted into a graphical and numerical mode in three ellipses where the area and the measurements of each ellipse include different percentages of fixation points (68.2%, 95.4%, and 99.6%) corresponding respectively to 1–2–3 standard deviations. The BCEA is expressed in square degrees, the major and minor axes are expressed in degrees, and the inclination of the major axis is expressed from −90° to 90° with 0° for the horizontal position.

The normal value of BCEA is 0.5–1° squared.

In audio-biofeedback, the pattern used for rehabilitation training is a chessboard format with six alternating schemes with varying radius, frequency in Hertz (number of pattern image changes in each second), and degrees of retinal coverage from 2° to 8° with elements of 0.5° in size or more.

Patients are trained to fix the new area of the retina by asking them to move their gaze toward the new fixation. As the patient moves, an intermittent sound plays. The closer the patient gets to the new zone, the more the sound will be continuous.

2.2 Case 1

A 73-year-old woman presented with neovascular AMD treated with intravitreal anti-vascular endothelial growth factor therapy (anti-VEGF) in both eyes.

Best corrected visual acuity (BCVA) in the right eye was 20/400, and BCVA in the left eye was 20/500.

Microperimetry MP1 Nidek showed a spontaneous and unstable PRL localized below compared to atrophic fovea with a medium sensitivity of 8 dB in the right eye (**Figure 1**). The eccentricity of fixation measured by microperimetry was 4° (**Figure 2**). The PRL area represented by the BCEA was 111.28° squared (3 Std Dev) (**Figure 3**).

The left eye with a worse visual functioning situation showed a spontaneous PRL located below and nasally with a medium sensitivity of 7 dB (**Figure 4**).

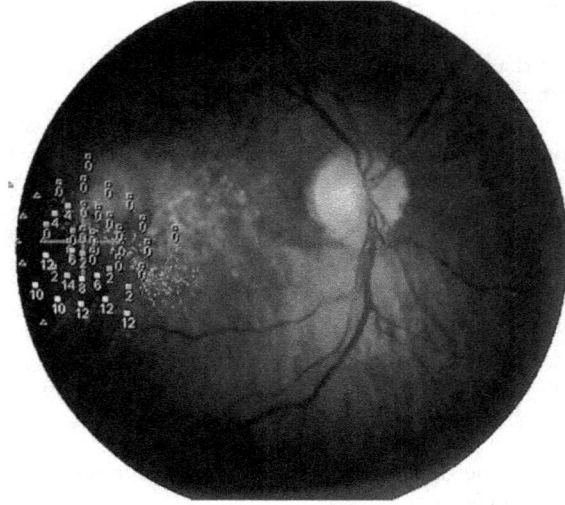

Figure 1.
Microperimetry before rehabilitation.

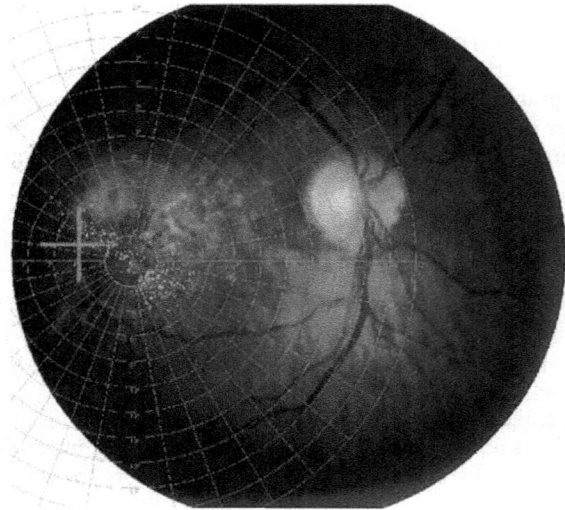

Figure 2.
Decentering of fixation before audio-biofeedback.

The eccentricity of fixation was 6° (**Figure 5**) and BCEA was 71.89° squared (**Figure 6**).

The patient completed 10 sessions of audio-biofeedback lasting 10 minutes per eye. After the audio-biofeedback, there was an improvement in the quality of vision.

The best corrected visual acuity (BCVA) in the right eye improved from 20/400 to 20/200, and in the left eye it improved from 20/500 to 20/400. The contrast sensitivity and the parameters of microperimetry improved as well. In the right eye, the PRL shifted from below to the temporal position with an increase of mean sensitivity from 8 dB to 13 dB (**Figure 7**).

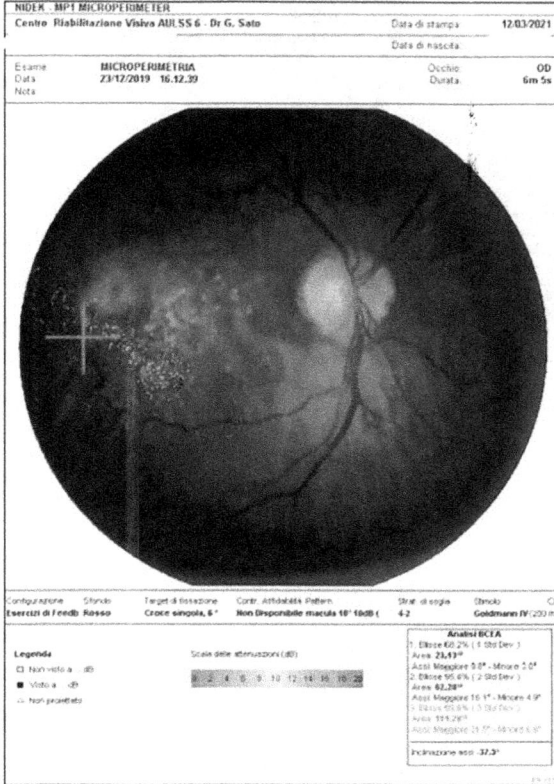

Figure 3.
BCEA before audio-biofeedback.

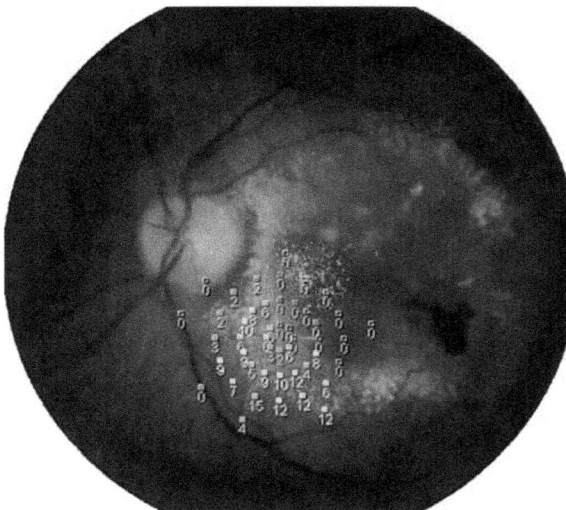

Figure 4.
PRL and mean sensitivity.

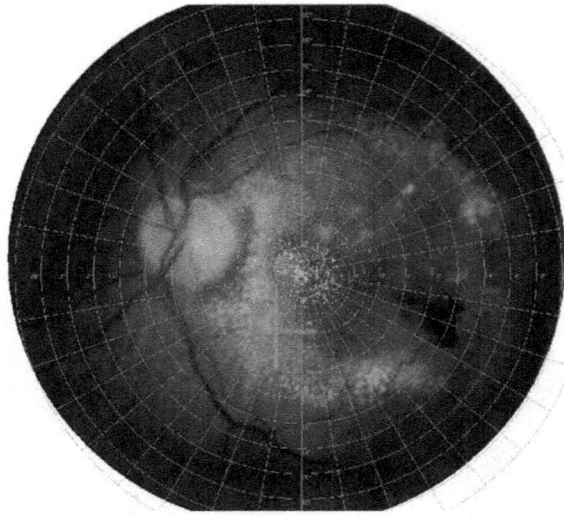

Figure 5.
Decentralization of fixation.

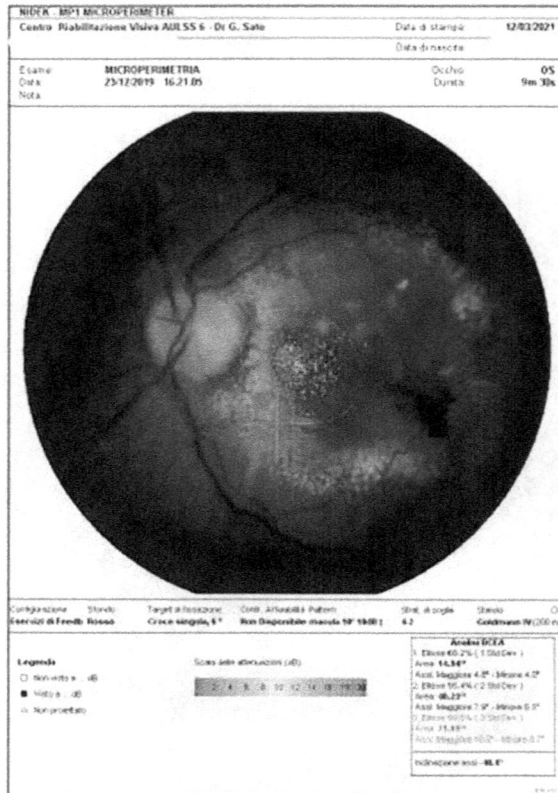

Figure 6.
BCEA before audio-bofeedback.

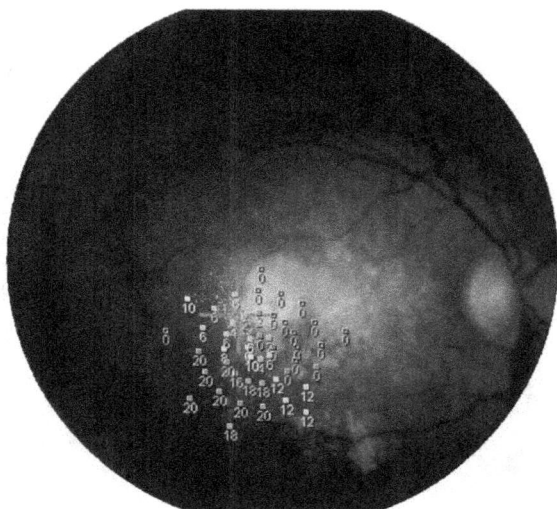

Figure 7.
In the RE the PRL shifted from below in temporal position.

The BCEA (bivariate contour ellipse area) decreased from 111.28° squared (3 st SD) to 31.12° squared, thus showing a clear improvement of fixation stability that is closely related to the improvement in mean sensitivity and to the shift of the PRL (**Figure 8**).

Beyond improvement in visual acuity, contrast sensitivity, stability of fixation, and sensitivity, as well as relocated fixation, the patient acquired the awareness of his own ability to fix, to use the visual residual, and to move toward the best site of vision (**Figure 9**).

2.3 Case 2

A 68-year-old woman presented with atrophic AMD. BCVA in both the right eye and left eye was 20/400.

The first microperimetry showed a central scotoma with a sensitivity of 0 dB without presence of PRL in the right eye but of an erratic searching of the presented fixation point without a precise point of fixation (**Figure 10**).

The BCEA area was 314.87° squared, and it was not possible to find the decentralization of fixation for the absence of fixation (**Figure 11**).

Microperimetry showed an unstable and spontaneous PRL located below the atrophic fovea with a mean sensitivity of 8 dB in the left eye (**Figure 12**).

The BCEA in the left eye was 90.10° squared (**Figure 13**).

The decentralization of fixation compared to the atrophic fovea was 7° (**Figure 14**).

The patient completed 10 sessions of audio-biofeedback in both eyes.

The purpose of the audio-biofeedback was to move the fixation up. In the right eye with erratic fixation, the cross was placed above the atrophic fovea, instead in the left eye the cross was placed above compared to the spontaneous PRL, which was located below the atrophic fovea (**Figure 15**). The passage from erratic fixation to superior fixation occurred gradually (**Figure 16**).

In the right eye, the fixation was shifted above and the sensitivity increased from 0 dB in the initial central scotoma with erratic fixation to 10 dB of mean sensitivity

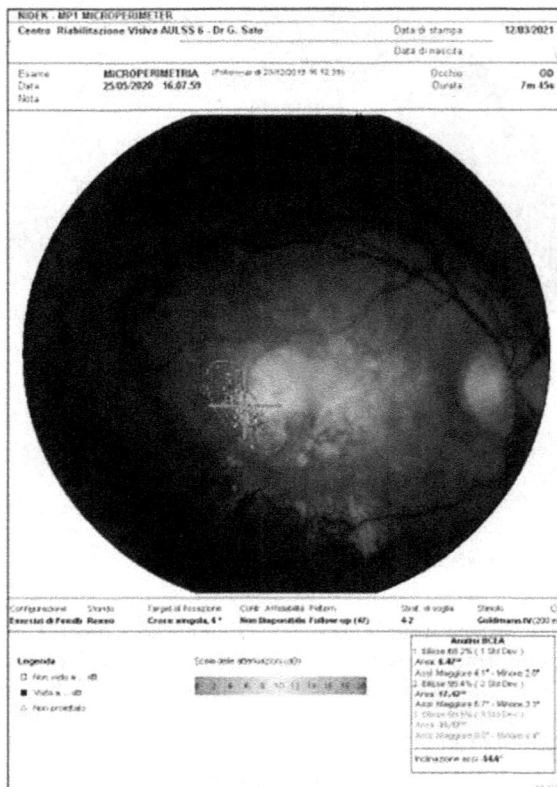

Figure 8.
Reduction of BCEA after ABFB with an increase in stability of the fixation.

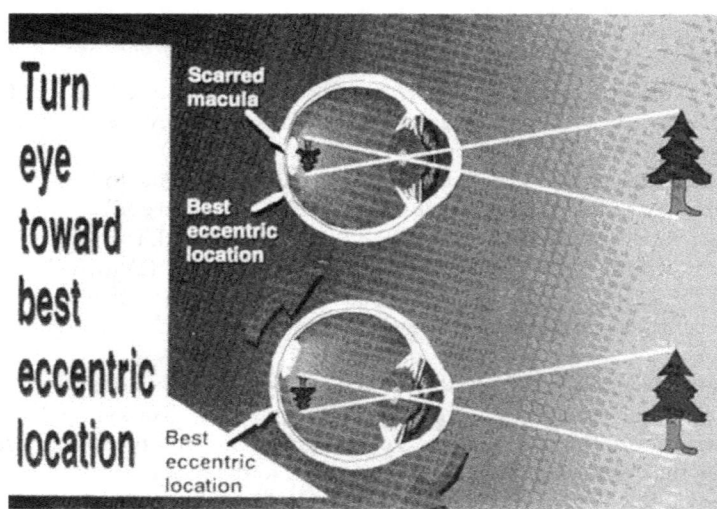

Figure 9.
The ocular movement toward the best eccentric fixation area allows the visually impaired patient with maculopathy to be able to see the tree.

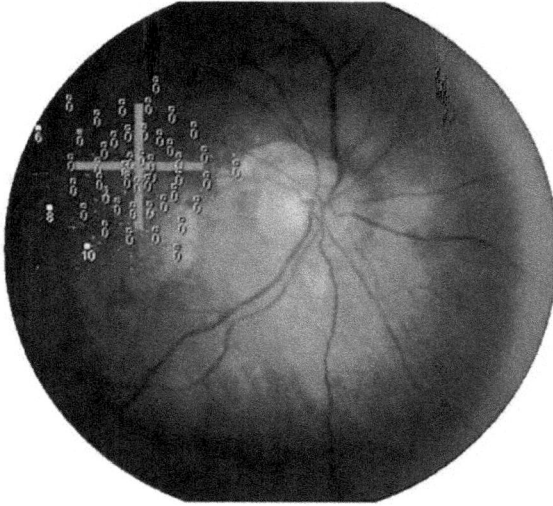

Figure 10.
RE: Erratic fixation.

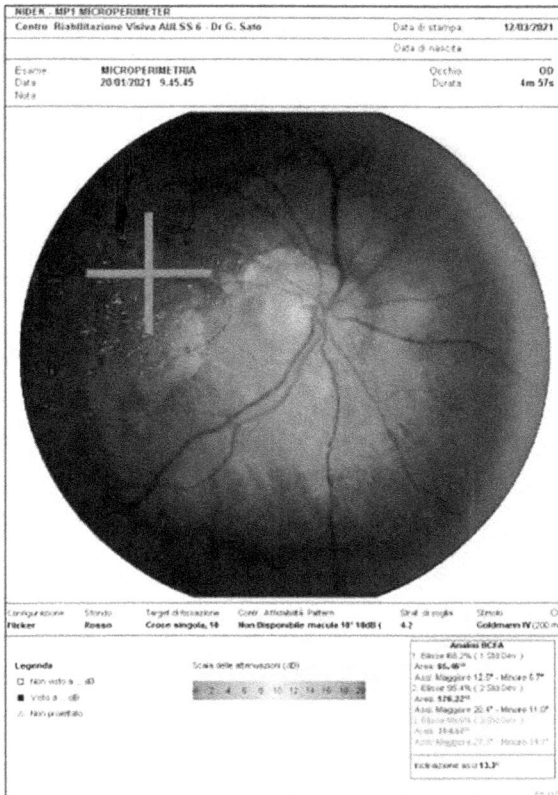

Figure 11.
RE: BCEA 314.87° squared.

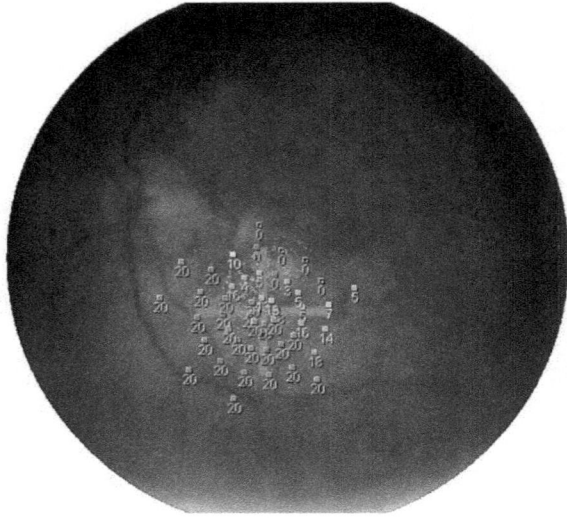

Figure 12.
Unstable and spontaneous PRL located below the atrophic fovea.

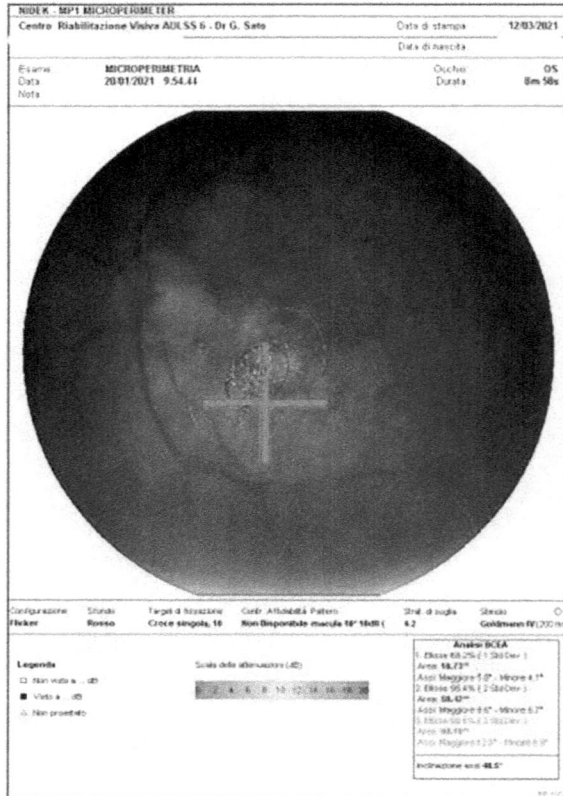

Figure 13.
BCEA 90.10° squared.

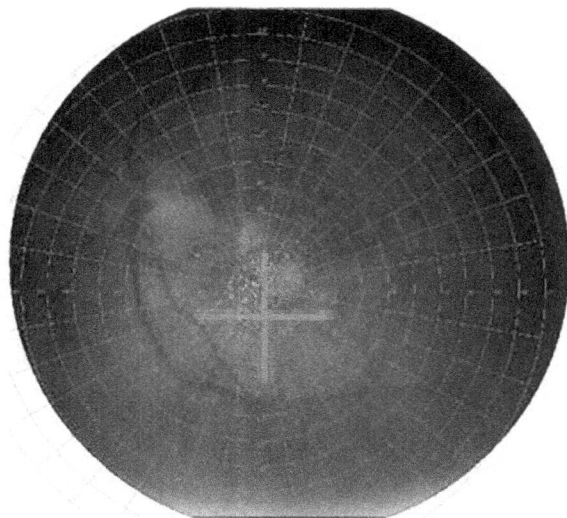

Figure 14.
Decentralization of eccentric fixation of 7°.

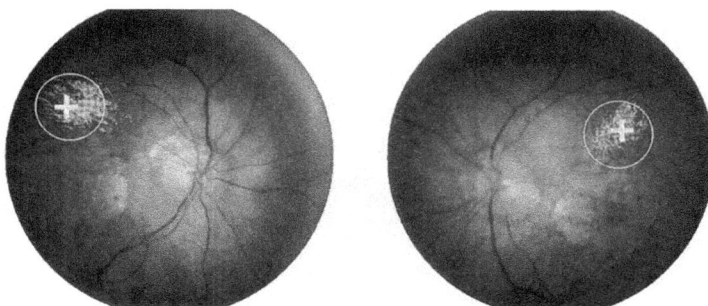

Figure 15.
Positioning of the best eccentric fixation in both eyes above the atrophic fovea.

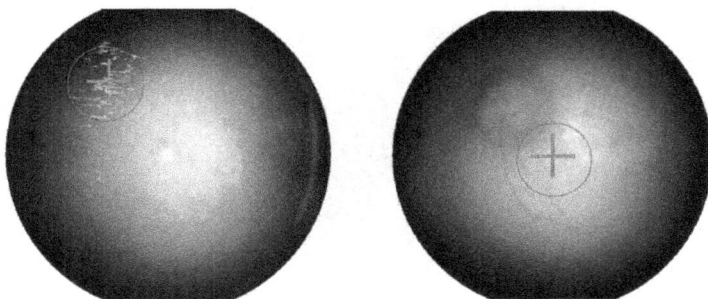

Figure 16.
Gradual shifting of fixation toward the best site of vision.

with the formation of a new area of fixation called the trained retinal locus (TRL) (**Figure 17**).

The BCEA in the new fixation, named TRL, was 144.24° squared (**Figure 18**) against 314.87° squared before the audio-biofeedback.

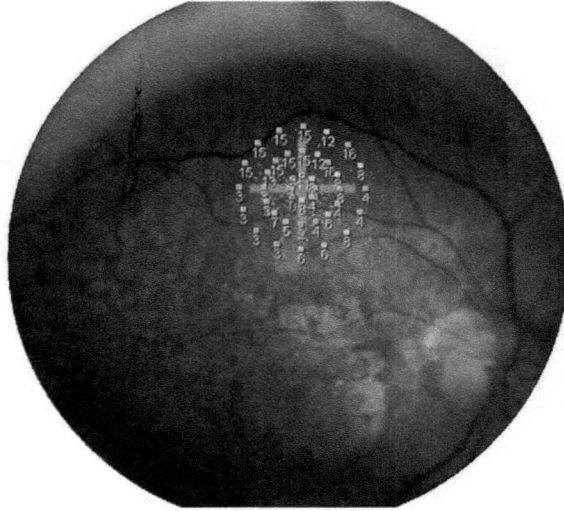

Figure 17.
RE: In the new trained fixation (TRL), the sensitivity is 10 dB.

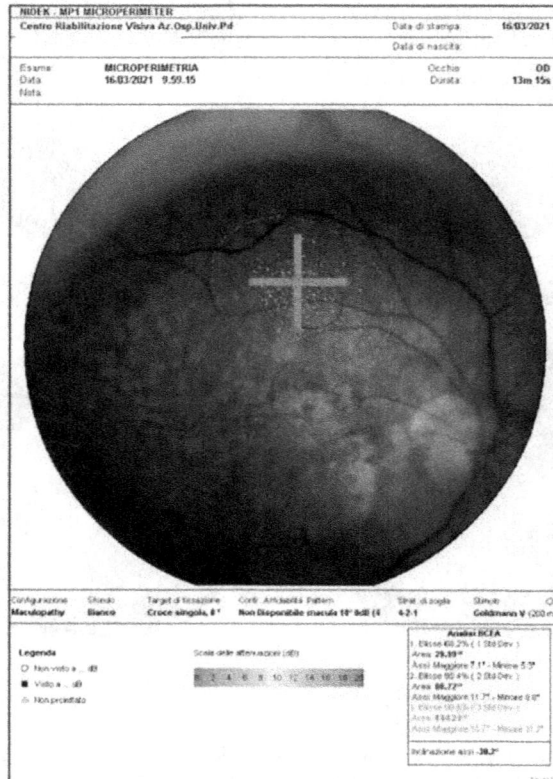

Figure 18.
RE: BCEA (bivariate contour ellipse area) after audio-biofeedback.

After ABFB, the visual acuity improved to 20/200 in both eyes and contrast sensitivity on the Pelli Robson chart increased from 0.60 to 0.90.

2.4 Case 3

A 67-year-old woman presented with AMD. Visual acuity in the right eye was finger count of 20 cm. Visual acuity in the left eye was 20/400 with visual disability. The patient was unable to read and cannot see faces. She was also unable to walk alone without serious problems in orientation and mobility.

Microperimetry showed an erratic fixation without a precise localization with central absolute scotoma and a sensitivity of 0.1 dB (**Figure 19**).

BCEA in the right eye was 185.08° squared in an erratic fixation (**Figure 20**).

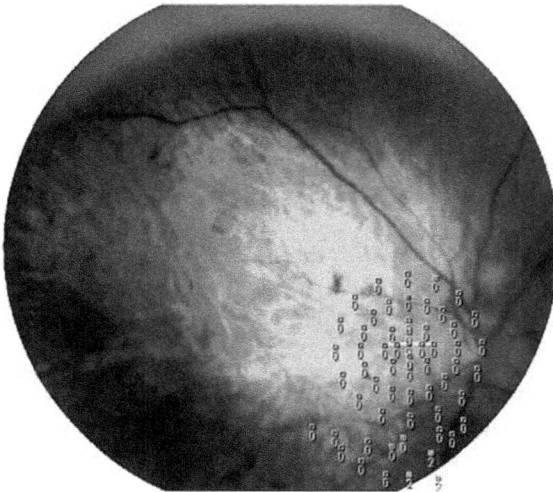

Figure 19.
RE: Erratic fixation.

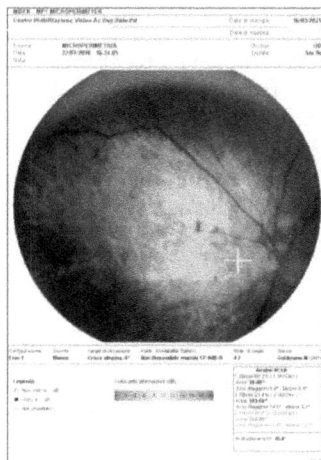

Figure 20.
RE: BCEA 185.08° squared in erratic fixation.

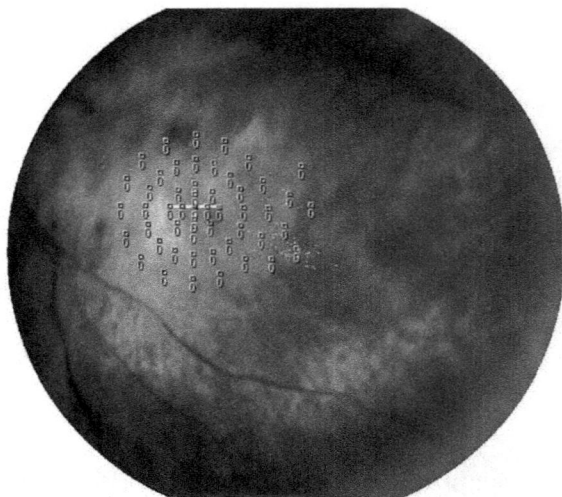

Figure 21.
LE: Absolute central scotoma.

In the left eye, there was a central absolute scotoma with a sensitivity of 0.00 dB (**Figure 21**).

BCEA in the left eye was 192.82° squared (**Figure 22**).

After 10 sessions of audio-biofeedback, we obtained a shift of the erratic fixation in a new PRL, named TRL, localized inferiorly to the optic disk near the very large atrophic maculopathy, extended beyond the posterior pole, with a sensitivity of 0.7 dB instead of 0.1 dB at the start. The sensitivity of the retina in the new area of fixation reached a good value of intensity until 10 dB (**Figure 23**).

In the new area of fixation, the BCEA was 73.39° squared (**Figure 24**).

In the left eye, after audio-biofeedback, we obtained a new area of fixation in the same site of the right eye, below the optic disk and near the large atrophic macular degeneration with a sensitivity of 0.5 dB from the initial absence in the central absolute scotoma (**Figure 25**).

The BCEA of the new TRL was 99.6° squared (**Figure 26**).

Visual acuity in the right eye improved from finger count to 20/400. Visual acuity in the left eye improved from 20/400 to 20/250. Before rehabilitation, the patient was not able to read with electronic aid. After ABFB, she was able to read with CCTV. Furthermore, she was able to see more clearly when walking, see the number of days of months in the calendar without glasses, and look at photos of family members. When she was able to see her father's photo, she was moved!

Often in low-vision rehabilitation, we find a PRL localized very far from the atrophic fovea (**Figures 27** and **28**).

In other cases, the PRL may be closer to the atrophic fibrotic fovea (**Figure 29**).

Still, in other cases, a very unstable foveal fixation must be stabilized (**Figure 30**).

In this case, we used a custom target of fixation with a four-word phrase that the patient can read when presented in the best area of fixation.

Figures 31 and **32** are examples of chessboard patterns used for audio-biofeedback.

Audio-biofeedback may be applied in other types of maculopathies such as hereditary retinal dystrophy, Stargardt disease, cone dystrophy, Best maculopathy, and myopic degeneration (**Figures 33–36**).

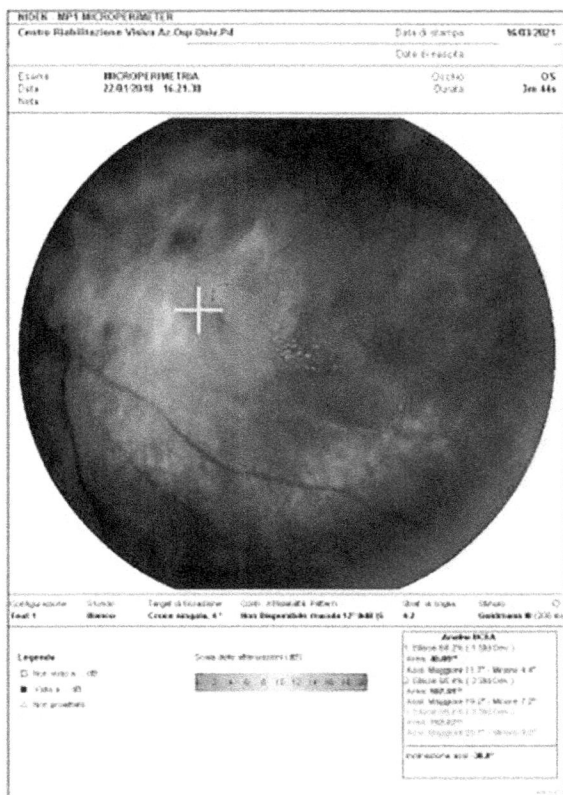

Figure 22.
LE: BCEA 192.82° squared.

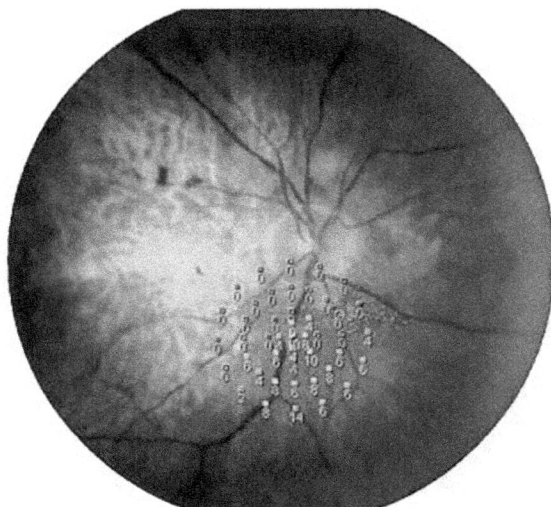

Figure 23.
RE: Trained retinal locus localized inferiorly to the optic disk with a sensitivity of 0.7 dB instead of 0.1 dB before audio-biofeedback in the erratic fixation.

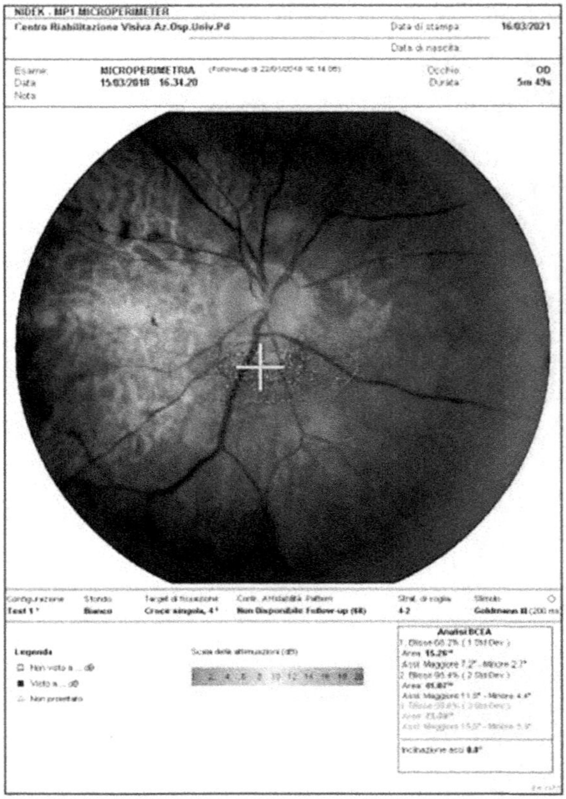

Figure 24.
RE: BCEA 73.39° squared instead 185.08° squared before audio-biofeedback.

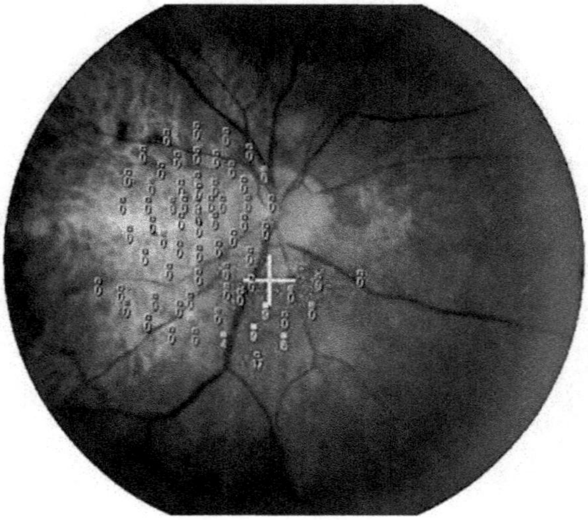

Figure 25.
LE: Trained retinal locus localized below the optic disk.

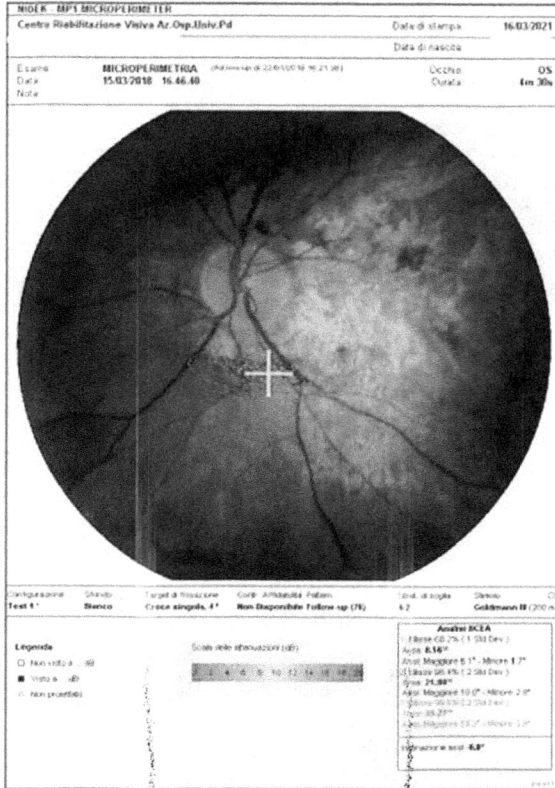

Figure 26.
In the new trained eccentric fixation, the BCEA decreased from 192.82° squared to 99.6° squared.

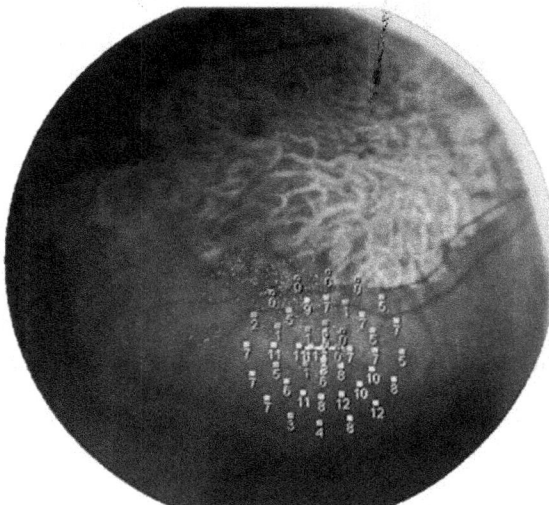

Figure 27.
Atrophic AMD with PRL located up in both eyes and very far from atrophic fovea.

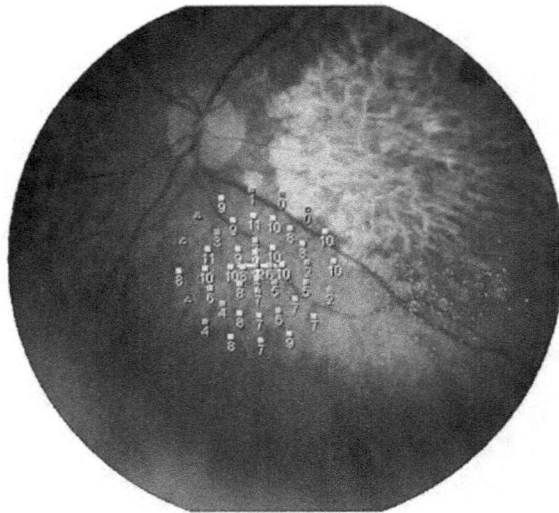

Figure 28.
Atrophic AMD with PRL located down in both eyes and very far from atrophic fovea.

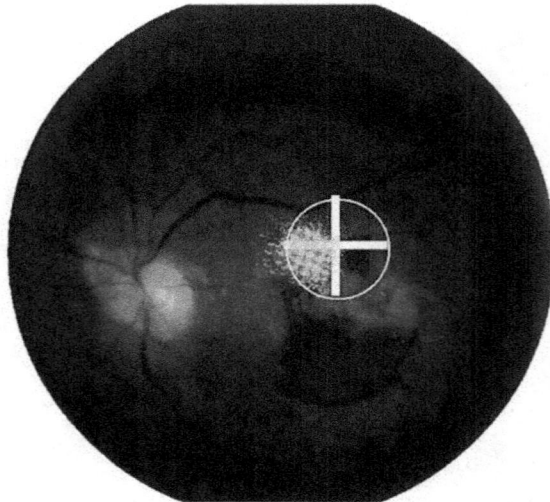

Figure 29.
PRL located up from atrophic fovea.

3. Conclusions

The improvements of retinal sensitivity in the new area of fixation (TRL) go hand in hand with an improvement in the quality of vision and the quality of life. Before low-vision rehabilitation with audio-biofeedback, the visually impaired patient is submitted to the Italian version of the Veterans Affairs (VA) Low-Vision Visual Functioning Questionnaire (LV VFQ-48) [8] based on the idea of Stelmack JA et al. [9] and with the permission of the authors. LV VFQ-48 is a fundamental instrument for measuring the difficulty low-vision persons have in performing daily activities and evaluating vision rehabilitation outcomes.

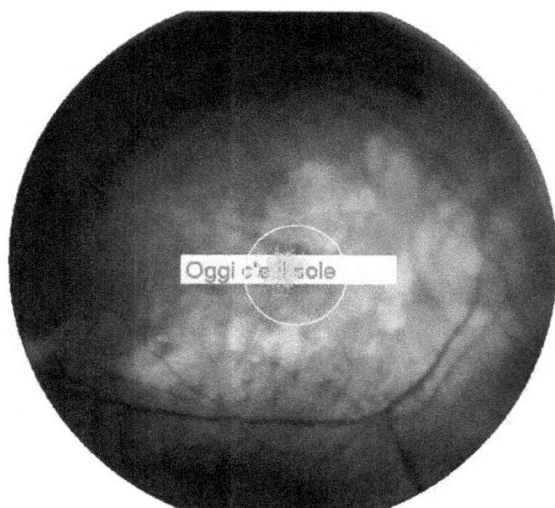

Figure 30.
Stabilization of fixation.

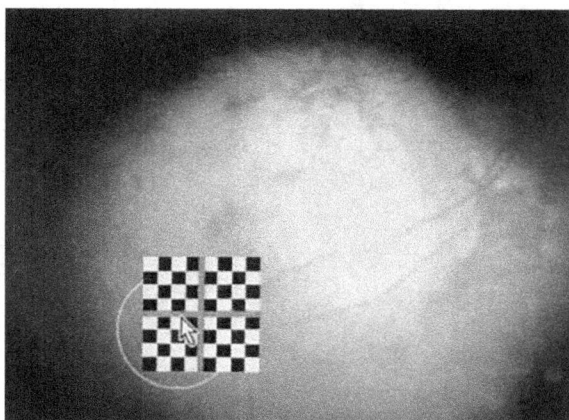

Figure 31.
Example of chessboard pattern used for audio-biofeedback.

After rehabilitation with audio-biofeedback, there was a positive change in the score regarding better vision in activities of daily living.

The chessboard pattern has an alternating reversal presentation. This leads to a neuro-visual stimulation of retina cells and consequently to a stimulation of the visual cortex with a cerebral reorganization based on the new occipital projection of the new PRL, which replaces the nonfunctioning macula [10, 11].

In conclusion, audio-biofeedback can stabilize the PRL with increased retinal sensitivity and improvement in BCEA, represented by a decrease in the fixation area. It can also lead to the development of a new area of fixation called the trained retinal locus (TRL).

Audio-biofeedback contributes to the patient's awareness of "where to look to see better." As such, ABFB for low-vision rehabilitation can improve both the quality of vision and the quality of life.

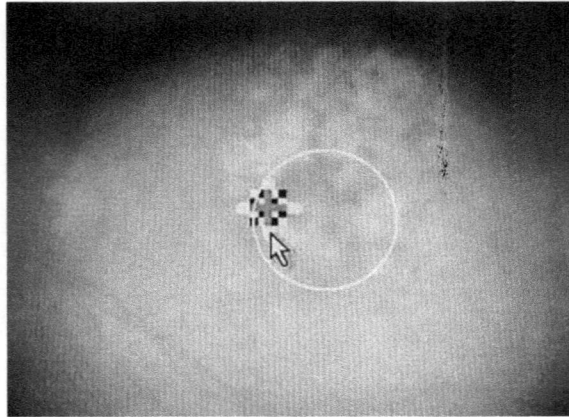

Figure 32.
Example of chessboard pattern used for audio-biofeedback.

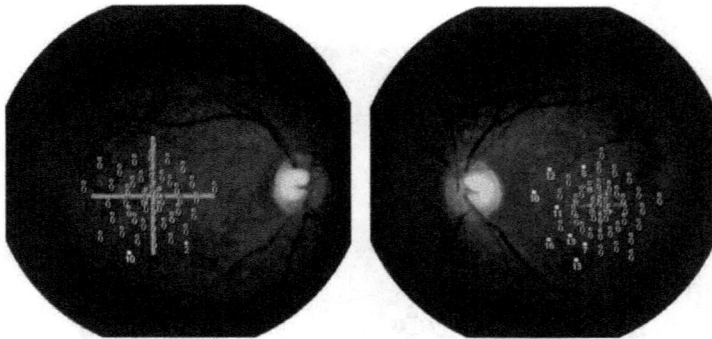

Figure 33.
Stargardt disease before audio-biofeedback.

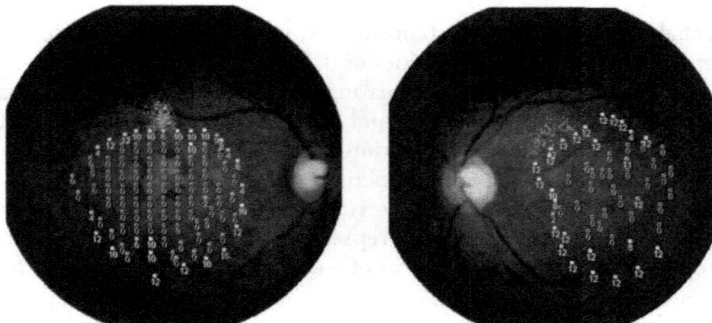

Figure 34.
Microperimetry in Stargardt disease after audio-biofeedback.

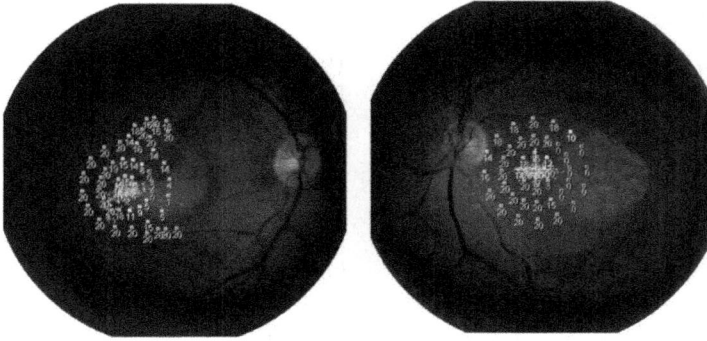

Figure 35.
Microperimetry in best disease after audio-biofeedback.

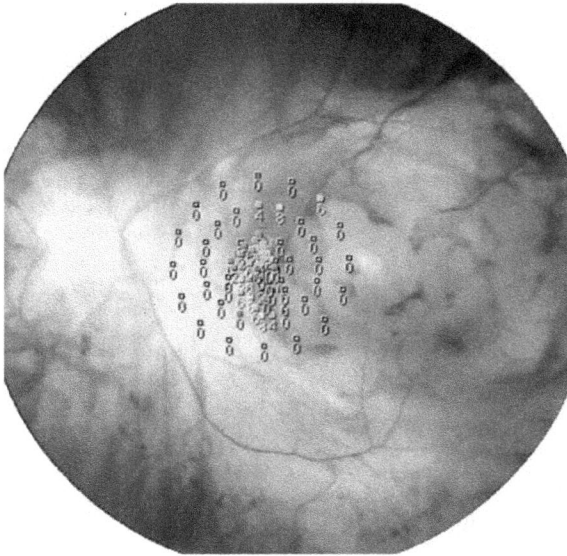

Figure 36.
Myopic macular degeneration.

Author details

Giovanni Sato* and Roberta Rizzo
Low Vision Rehabilitation Center – Azienda Ospedale – Università, Padova, Italy

*Address all correspondence to: giovanni.sato@aopd.veneto.it

IntechOpen

References

[1] Epstein LH, Blanchar EB. Biofeedback self-control and self management. Biofeedback Self Regulation. 1977;2(2):201-211

[2] Giggins OM, Persson UM, Caulfield B. Biofeedback in rehabilitation. Journal of Neuroengineering Rehabilitation. Jun 2013;18:10-60

[3] Vingolo EM, Cavarretta S, Domanico D, Parisi F, Malagola R. Microperinetric biofeedback in AMD patients. Applied Psychophysiology Biofeedback. 2007;32(3–4):185-189

[4] Crossland MD, Dunbar HM, Rubin GS. Fixation stability measurement using the MP1 microperimeter. Retina. 2009;29: 651-656

[5] Markowitz SN, Reyes SV. Microperimetry and clinical practise: An evidence based review. Canadian Journal of Ophthalmology. 2013;48(5): 350-357

[6] Fujii GY, De Juan E, Humayun MS, Sunness JS, Chang TS, Rossi JV. Characteristics of visual loss by scanning laser ophthalmoscope microperimetry in eyes with subfoveal choroideal neovascolarization secondary to age related macular degeneration. American Journal of Ophthalmology. 2003;136(6):1067-1078

[7] Timberlake GT, Sharma MK, Grose SA, Gobert DV, Gauch JM, Maino JH. Retinal location of the preferred retinal locus relative to the fovea in scanning laser ophthalmoscope images. Optometry Vision Science. 2005;82(3):177-185

[8] Di Maggio I, Virgili G, Giacomelli G, Murro V, Sato G, Amore F, et al. The veterans affairs low-vision visual functioning Questionnaire-48 (VA LV VFQ-48): Performance of the Italian version. European Journal of Ophthalmology. 2020;30(5):1014-1018

[9] Stelmack JA, Szlyk JP, Stelmack TR, Demers-Turco P, Williams RT, Moran D, et al. Measuring outcomes of low vision rehabilitation with vision visual funnstioning questionnaire. Investigative Ophthalmology Vision Science. 2006;47(8):3253-3261

[10] Vingolo EM, Napolitano G, Fragiotta S. Microperimetric biofeedback training: Fundamentals, strategies and perspectives. Frontiers in Bioscience Scholar. 2018;10:48-64

[11] Baker CI, Peli E, Knouf N, Kanwisher NG. Reorganization of visual processing in macular degeneration. Journal of Neuroscience. 2005;25(3): 614-618

Evidence-Based Practice and Trends in Visual Rehabilitation for Patients with Age-Related Macular Degeneration

Luis Leal Vega, Irene Alcoceba Herrero,
Adrián Martín Gutiérrez, Joaquín Herrera Medina,
Natalia Martín Cruz, Juan F. Arenillas Lara
and María Begoña Coco Martín

Abstract

Age-related macular degeneration (AMD) is a common, chronic, and progressive eye disease that is considered the leading cause of visual loss among the elderly in developed countries. Advanced AMD, including choroidal neovascularization (CNV) or geographic atrophy (GA), is associated with substantial and progressive visual impairment that can lead to a significant reduction in functional independence and quality of life (QoL) for affected individuals, whose number is expected to increase in the coming years in line with population growth and ageing. In this context, while an important part of medical care is focused on preventing the progression of the disease, Visual Rehabilitation (VR) aims to address its consequences by providing these patients with a number of strategies to achieve their goals and participate autonomously, actively and productively in society. This chapter aims to provide an update on evidence-based practices in the field and how modern technologies play an important role in the development of new VR approaches.

Keywords: age-related macular degeneration, visual rehabilitation, management, technology, practice, trends

1. Introduction

Age-related macular degeneration (AMD) is a prevalent, progressive eye disease that is characterized by a late-onset neuro-degeneration of the photoreceptors (light-sensitive retinal cells) and their supporting tissues [1].

It is considered a highly disabling disease, as the macula (part of the eye responsible for sharp, clear vision) is the most damaged area of the retina, causing a gradual loss of central vision with subsequent difficulties in many activities of daily living (ADLs) for those affected, such as reading, driving, mobility or face recognition.

Globally, AMD is responsible for approximately 7% of blindness and 3% of visual impairment, making it the third most common cause of vision loss worldwide, and the first in industrialized countries [2, 3].

In economic terms, the total cost due to AMD is estimated to be approximately $343 billion, including $255 billion in direct healthcare costs (due to scheduled medical visits, treatment, rehabilitation, vision-related equipment, etc.) and $88 billion in indirect costs (due to injury, depression, loss of productivity, and social dependence as a consequence of blindness caused by the disease) [4]. Furthermore, the progressive growth and ageing of the population suggests that the magnitude of this issue will increase in the coming years, with the global prevalence of AMD expected to rise from 199 million people in 2020 to 288 million in 2040 [5].

From a clinical perspective, AMD can be classified into early and late stages. Patients with early AMD are usually asymptomatic and present yellowish drusen and pigmentary alterations in the macular area on fundus examination (**Figure 1**), while late stages of the disease, responsible for most visual loss attributed to AMD, are defined by the presence of signs indicating choroidal neovascularization (CNV) or geographic atrophy (GA) [6].

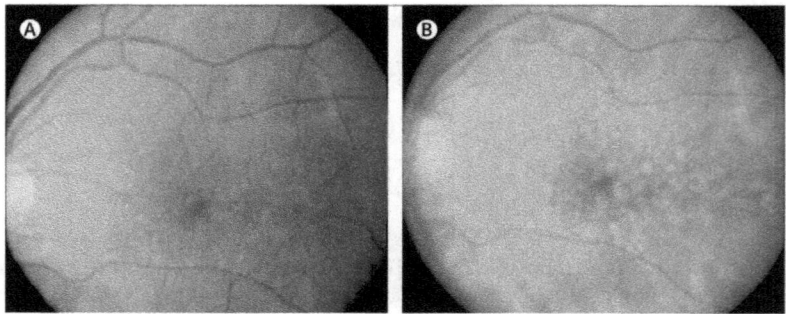

Figure 1.
Large drusen appearing as yellowish subretinal spots present in a patient with early AMD from the Blue Mountains Eye Study [7] (A) and progression of both drusen size and area involved over 5 years (B) [6].

In CNV (wet) AMD, abnormal blood vessels grow and break through to the neural retina (**Figure 2**). These new blood vessels are fragile and tend to leak blood, fluid and lipids, which can accumulate under the macular area, elevating it and distorting vision and eventually leading to the formation of fibrous scarring.

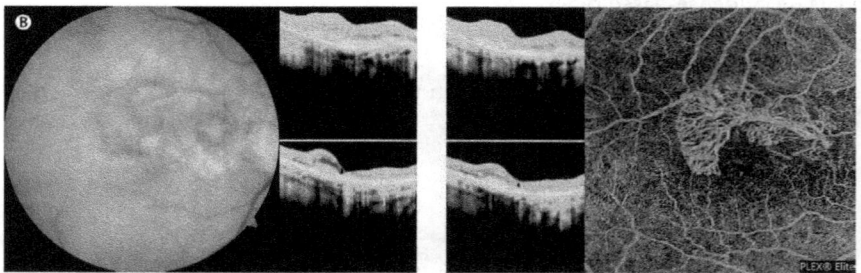

Figure 2.
Recent-onset neovascular AMD on colour photography (left), spectral-domain optical coherence tomography (middle), and optical coherence tomography angiography showing appearance of choroidal new vessels (right) [8].

On the other hand, in atrophic (late dry) AMD, a gradually deterioration of the retinal pigmentary epithelium (RPE), choriocapillaris, and photoreceptors occurs (**Figure 3**). As both AMD forms progresses, detail in front of central visual field is lost and over time a blind spot (scotoma) may appear in the central visual field of the patient [8].

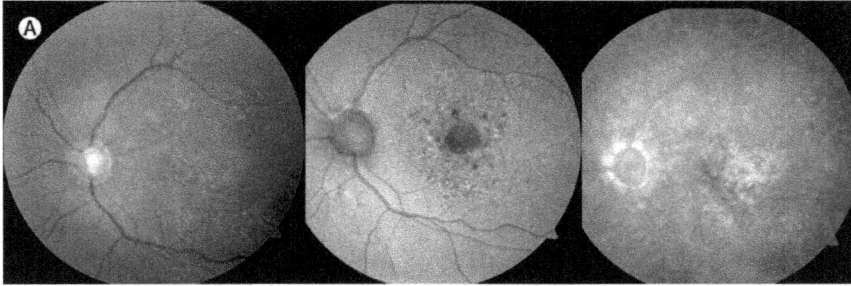

Figure 3.
Large soft drusen surrounding an area of GA on colour fundus photography (left), fundus autofluorescence imaging (middle), and fluorescein angiography (right) [8].

Although the initial cause of AMD remains unclear, several risk factors have been linked to the development of the disease, such as age (>60 years), lifestyle (smoking, diet), cardiovascular disease and genetic markers [9].

This suggest that the pathogenesis of AMD is the result of a complex multi-factorial interaction between environmental, functional, genetic and metabolic factors involving multiple biological pathways, including inflammation, angio-genesis, remodeling of the extracellular matrix, lipid metabolism and transport regulation, etc. [10–12].

In recent years, several epidemiological studies have reported a decrease in blindness and visual impairment associated with AMD [13, 14], which is likely to be attributed to improved diagnostic procedures, earlier diagnosis, slowing disease progression through micronutrient supplementation [15, 16], and the introduction of new therapies based on suppression of vascular endothelial growth factor (VEGF) [17].

Unfortunately, despite all this progress in AMD management, there is currently no effective treatment to cure the disease or reverse its course. However, in most patients, peripheral vision is preserved, allowing them to retain a certain level of autonomy.

On this basis, visual rehabilitation (VR) aims to provide these people with a range of strategies and behaviors to achieve the full potential of their remaining vision, improving their self-confident and independence and enabling them to return to a visually active life as much as possible. This philosophy aims at increasing awareness in low-vision patients, so they do not just focus on their loss or their impairment.

2. Visual rehabilitation as part of AMD care

People who do not have AMD (e.g., family members, caregivers, and even some healthcare providers) often underestimate the effect of this condition, particularly in terms of visual function and quality of life (QoL) [18].

According to the World Health Organization' (WHO), disability must include both the impairment of bodily structures or functions and the difficulty or limitation in performing a task and in participating in life situations [19].

This approach implies that the rehabilitation process cannot only focus on the aspects that directly affect the person, but must also deal with the society in which they live and the context that makes it possible for them to develop, in order to have a successful life.

Paying attention to this, comprehensive AMD care should give attention not only to the structural and functional condition of the eye, but also to the patient's functioning in his or her specific surrounding. In this sense, the main difference between VR and other ophthalmic sub-specialties is that most of these sub-specialties are anatomically defined, while VR is functionally defined (**Figure 4**) [20].

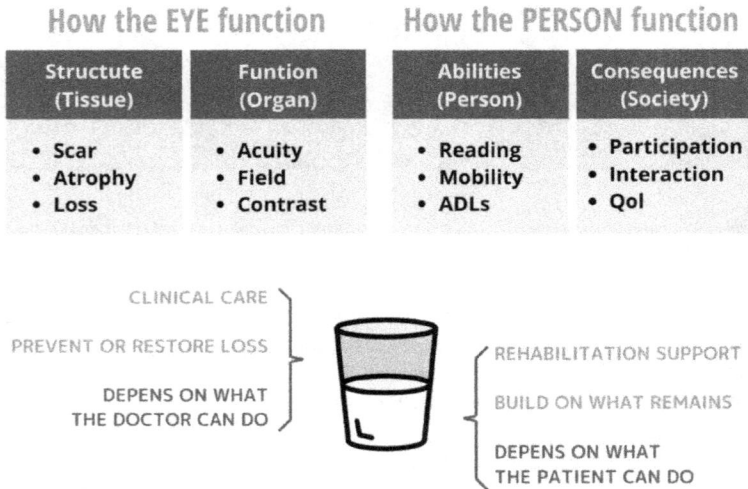

Figure 4.
Comprehensive AMD care diagram showing the areas of influence and differences between medical and rehabilitative care. Adapted from: [20].

To adequately cover all these aspects, the participation and collaboration of different professionals is necessary, since different goals often require different interventions [21]. This can be observed in the US and Europe models, where a wide range of professionals, varying from continent to continent, work together to achieve a successful rehabilitation.

Multidisciplinary low-vision teams usually require an ophthalmology, an optometrist, an occupational therapist and a rehabilitation teacher among other professionals specially trained in the evaluation of the patient's remaining vision and the prescription of different low-vision aids (LVAs) [22]. However, prescription of these aids is only the first step in learning how to use them effectively, as training and continuous practice are essential to help the patient feel comfortable and get the most out of them [23]. To this end, different techniques can be employed, often using both office- and home-based exercises with the device while performing a specific activity for a few hours in different sessions [24–26].

Besides prescription of LVAs and training on their correct use, VR also con-templates assessment of the home environment, as well as psychological and social worker support. Despite this, it should not be ignored that, according to the Veterans Affairs Low Vision Intervention Trial II (LOVIT II), basic low vision services are sufficient for most people with low vision, although basic services combined with VR programs are most effective for people with a visual acuity of 20/200 or less [27].

3. Visual rehabilitation for AMD patients

VR in AMD patients has largely focused on reading [28] and for this purpose many LVAs have been used. But, today, individuals with AMD demand wider objectives that include, apart for reading, being able to participate in other activities and carry out their daily life and travels independently. If we add to this the fact that modern technologies have greatly expanded access to information for people with low-vision, we get that VR encompass a variety of resources to ultimately fit the person's goals, needs and demands.

Reading is a sophisticated activity of great importance for the life of the individual in its personal, educational or professional aspects. Conditions compromising the condition of the macula, such as AMD, can greatly affect this ability, which adequate performance largely depends on the reception of central visual information. Depending on the degree to which the scotoma is affected, the reading speed in these patients can be between 25 and 130 words per minute (wpm), while the average reading speed of a person without visual impairment is usually around 200-250 wpm [29].

In everyday life, everyone needs to be able to read texts whose size covers a range from newspaper print to headlines. People with normal vision perform this task with a speed that favors comprehension and comfort. However, AMD patients find that reading speed is compromised as the font size becomes smaller. In general, this population needs magnification of the text to achieve a reading speed that allows them to read effectively, although this will always be lower than that of people without AMD.

In individuals with central field loss (CFL), eccentric fixation is necessary, and the oculomotor pattern differs when reading. Eye movements in people with severe visual impairment tend towards continuous refixation, i.e., fixation stability is weak, and not always stable and functional [30]. Consequently, letter recognition is slower and more difficult [31]. Sometimes, it is difficult to recognize a word with a single fixation, being necessary several saccades within the same word [32]. Visual field loss close to fixation can also affect everyday activities, such as face recognition or shopping [33].

With this in mind, most functional adaptations in these cases are based on training in the use of a preferred retinal locus (PRL) to make eye movements remain in a functional area of the peripheral retina. This PRL is empowered to assume the macular function and thus restore the lost vision-related skills, so assessing its location and characteristics is an essential part of any reading rehabilitation program [34]. In this context, microperimeters offer the most accurate method for PRL assessment (**Figure 5**).

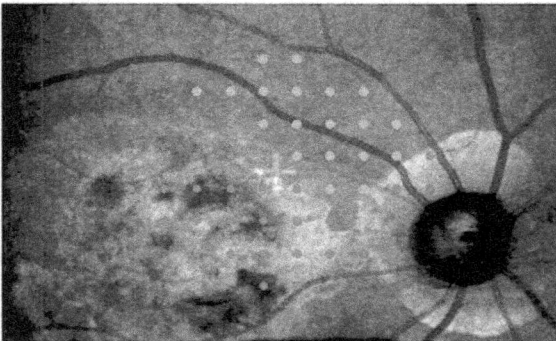

Figure 5.
Microperimetry using a standard grid (52 points) in a study of ranibizumab effects on functional vision in patients with advanced AMD [35] showing the non-visual area of the retina (red points), the normal sensitive retina (green points) and the patient's fixation target (cross) [36].

The subject's ability to make visual movements so that the target is held in the PRL correlates with reading speed, as do more intense saccadic movements and stability of fixation [37]. In addition to holding the target on the retina, the eye must move rapidly towards objects further away in the field of vision (saccadic movements). The angle at which the movement to fix the image in the PRL must be made will affect the fixation, the stability of which is crucial for reading and proper perception.

After eccentric viewing training, the location of the retinal area used for fixation may change, but not the fixation stability [38]. Moreover, the person does not always use the same PRL, and may use several depending on the target position. Some authors report that these PRLs may appear untrained in patients in the first six months of disease [38]. Many patients with AMD adopt an PRL on the left area of the scotoma, although more information is obtained from the right area during reading. For this reason, Rubin [39] suggests that it is preferable to use the right area of the scotoma to the left.

The benefits of eccentric viewing training on the reading performance of patients with AMD have been supported by several studies. For example, Nilsson et al. [40] trained 20 patients with neovascular AMD, an absolute central scotoma, and a mean best-corrected visual acuity (BCVA) of 20/475 in the use of a new and more favorable PRL for reading, observing that, after a mean training time of 5.2 hours, 90% of the participants learned to use eccentric viewing, which correlated with a significant improvement in reading speed from 9.0 ± 5.8 words per minute (wpm) to 68.3 ± 19.4 wpm.

A larger sample study evaluating the influence of eccentric viewing training in 242 individuals with a central scotoma concluded that, after an average training time of 3.8 hours, reading speed increased from 48.0 wpm to 71.9 wpm, the size of Arial font that could be read fluently could be reduced from 14.3 to 11.5, the duration of comfortable reading improved from 1.7 to 15.8 min, and the mean percentage of material that was understood by patients could be increased from 73.7 to 92.7% [41].

In addition, when compared with other interventions in the literature, such as a microperimetric biofeedback and microscope teaching program, eccentric viewing training has been found to offer greater benefit in terms of improved reading speed among patients with AMD [42].

It can be said that reading is significantly slower in patients who have not been trained in the use of the retinal locus, but, according to the findings of Watson et al., this does not mean that PRL training should not be further investigated [43].

But different oculomotor pattern is not the only factor that explains the lower reading speed in patients with macular degeneration. Cheong et al. concluded that in patients with AMD the visual processing of letter recognition is also lower, thus negatively influencing reading speed, reading comprehension and enjoyment while reading, as well as resistance in avoiding visual fatigue [44].

Another factor that can determine the efficiency of reading in patients with AMD is the number of characters that can be recognized in each fixation or visual span. This, in addition to the slower visual processing observed in these patients, forces more frequent eye movements. According to Chung [45], training can lengthen the visual lag in normal peripheral vision, although this benefit is less pronounced in older people.

For some researchers, contrast sensitivity is shown to be a critical factor in explaining the future reading efficiency of the patient with AMD over other factors such as scotoma size or BCVA [46]. In general, it can be said that individuals with AMD require contrast enhancement to achieve their optimal reading speed level [47, 48].

Lighting is another key component involved in the reading rehabilitation process for people with AMD, as the negative effect of uncontrolled illumination hinders vision. In this context, it is known that people with AMD often require high levels of illumination [49]. According to Bower et al., [50] at least 2000 lux are necessary to improve reading performance in patients with AMD, although Seiple et al. [51] indicate that this benefit can only be considered for small font sizes.

Finally, it should be pointed out that various studies have tried to establish the degree of importance the way the text is presented has on reading performance in AMD patients.

Chung is one of the researchers who has dedicated her work to this, although she states that there is not enough evidence that typography or text formatting (e.g., page formatting, Rapid Serial Visual Presentation: RSVP, scrolling text) improves reading speed, except in some cases of RSVP [52, 53]. In clinical practice, these are factors that may affect visual comfort and the subjective perception of improved reading or reduced visual fatigue differently from person to person.

4. Low vision aids for AMD patients

4.1 Non-optical aids

Environmental adaptations such as adequate illumination (by the use of light flexes or lecterns) and glare reduction and light with specific wavelengths preferred by the patients (by the use of prescription filters) are two well-known beneficial strategies for improving functional outcome measures in CFL patients.

These interventions result in apparent improved contrast sensitivity and better visual acuity for AMD patients [54, 55], so ensuring these optimal conditions is a fundamental step prior to the prescription of any additional aid.

Increasing the amount of light has demonstrated to have a significant positive effect on sentence reading acuity, reading speed and critical letter size for AMD patients [50].

In addition, some authors who have investigated the effects of making light adjustments in the homes of people with visual impairment have found that higher lighting levels led to greater well-being and a significant improvement in certain instrumental ADLs [56].

The use of filters has also been shown to improve vision-related QoL in patients with AMD, with the success rate of filter placement being better for those patients with visual acuity less than 0.25 and those with advanced AMD [57]. Nevertheless, although various tests exist to determine the best color, tint, lens material or frame type for a given patient, to date no specific protocol has been developed to assist in prescribing tinted or selective transmission lenses [58].

4.2 Optical aids

Optical aids for near vision involve the use of lenses to reduce the viewing distance of an object, making it easier to see, and are primarily used to tasks requiring near resolution acuity, such as reading, writing, personal care (i.e., make-up, nail polishing) and different leisure activities, such as sewing or drawing.

These optical LVAs broadly include the use of high-plus reading lenses and different magnifiers (including clip-on, hand-held, or stand devices), which power will ultimately depend on the patient's remaining vision and on the size of the object or printed material to be seen by the patient [59, 60]. In a consecutive sample of 100 individuals with AMD, these optical LVAs was shown to improve near BCVA from 0.13 (decimal) to 0.39 [61].

When reading with a hand-held magnifier, the magnifier has to move along the line and at the same time keep a constant distance from the text to ensure a clear image [62].

Clip-on magnifiers overcome this disadvantage, but can nevertheless scratch the lenses and reduce the visual field to further distances. In this context, stand magnifiers are the choice preferred by patients, as they offer ergonomic advantages such as a comfortable viewing angle, the possibility of both reading and writing, better illumination, a wider field of view, variable power and magnification, and a greater working distance [63].

Magnification can also be achieved with the use of telescopic devices, which are used to recognize objects that are outside the near vision range. These optical aids can be used for tasks such as reading street signs, road signs, and transport time-tables, making them a great ally for outdoor mobility. Furthermore, additional magnifying devices can easily be applied to these devices to improve near vision as well.

In recent years, advances in surgery have allowed intraocular implantation of these devices. Implantable miniature telescopes (IMTs) are visual prosthetic devices usually implanted monocularly depending on the eye with BCVA and, once implanted, are used to magnify objects in the patient's central visual field and focus them onto healthy areas of the retina, allowing them to recognize objects they would otherwise not be able to see [64]. In this way, the implanted eye is responsible for detailed vision, and the fellow eye will be responsible for peripheral vision tasks, including ambulation.

The safety and efficacy of these devices has been evaluated in different clinical trials that have found similar improvements in BCVA after one year of implantation ($\approx$60% of participants gained three or more lines in either distance or near BCVA), with no serious adverse events reported [65, 66]. In addition, a follow-up study showed that substantial visual improvements achieved with the intervention were maintained at two years [67].

4.3 Electronic aids

Electronic vision enhancement systems include closed-circuit television (CCTV) systems and other systems incorporating a monitor or a liquid-crystal display (LCD) screen in which the image or the print is projected after being digitized.

These systems provide increased magnification and an enlarged field of view than traditional optical aids, with the possibility of controlling relevant parameters, such as brightness, glare or contrast, so they can be appropriate for individuals which vision is greatly reduced or in which the use of optical aids have failed in achieving their goals.

For example, in a retrospective study of 530 patients with different stages of AMD in which participants were provided with different LVAs, successful VR (reading ability in 94% of patients when only 16% could read before) was achieved with optical visual aids in 58% of patients, whereas 42% needed electronic CCTV systems [68].

A clinical trial in which 37 subjects with central field loss were randomized to receive standard VR (group A = 18 subjects) or standard VR plus electronic magnifiers (group = 19 subjects) showed that, at 1 month, group B read faster and was better at two spot reading tasks such as reading continuous print and finding a number in a phone book, but did not differ from the group A in terms of functional capacity or well-being [69].

In another crossover study comparing the near vision activity performance of 84 experienced users of optical aids when using portable electronic vision enhancement systems plus optical magnifiers or optical magnifiers alone, it was observed that, at 2 months, the use of electronic systems allowed longer duration of reading. In addition, participants reported less difficulty performing a range of near vision activities when using these systems and were able to perform more tasks independently [70].

In addition to CCTV systems, these LVAs include the use of head-mounted displays (HMDs) [71], which enhance vision by coupling digital image processing directly to the patient's retina, and the use of portable electronic devices (such as tablets, smart-phones and electronic readers), which combine the portability of hand-held magnifiers with the high-resolution displays of electronic magnifiers (CCTV) and incorporate basic features for handling optical characteristics that can be useful to improve functional measures in patients with AMD, such as image enlargement or contrast polarity [72, 73].

5. Emerging trends in the field

Traditionally, VR in AMD patients includes training in eccentric vision and learning to use different optical and electronic magnifiers. However, some authors have recently studied the effects of new strategies, such as Barraza-Bernal et al. [74], who conducted a study with fifteen subjects with normal vision under simulation conditions, showing that PRL can be induced in a specific area by systematic relocation of stimuli.

Similarly, Morales et al. discuss improving the fixation stability in the PRL through biofeedback fixation training (BFT), which consist of slightly moving the gaze towards the training locus during different sessions [75]. Another training paradigm integrating oculomotor control and pattern recognition has also been evaluated, demonstrating that these strategies combined are capable of inducing a PRL over a short period of time in eight subjects with normal vision and a simulated central scotoma [76].

There are several studies that have been carried out to determine the effectiveness of repetitive, perceptual learning as an intervention approach for VR. This approach refers to the improvement in the execution of perceptual tasks as a consequence of training.

Perceptual learning has been found to have neural correlates in visual cortex, which declines with age. Learning effects in older adults are shown to be less than in younger people and are transferred only for the typeface and the retinal location trained. Causes may be a lower visual base span, decreased attention when exercising eccentricity, and less retention of what is learned over time.

People with AMD have a lower visual span, which contributes to a lower peripheral reading speed. According to Legge et al. [77], peripheral reading speed may improve if the size of the peripheral visual span is enlarged, and training based on letter-recognition trials has shown to extend the visual span, contributing to improve reading speed among older adults [78]. These studies [79] were carried out using trigrams, while Bernard et al. [80] sough to find out if a greater benefit can be obtained by using trigrams based on the most commonly used combinations in the English language, determining that the effects of perceptual learning may not be linked to the type of related letters.

Among several studies that have tried to determine the benefits of perpetual learning, some differentiate the way in which texts are presented. Among those using RSVP, there are differences between the vertical and horizontal presentation of text. For example, Yu et al. [81] found that lower speed in vertical presentation corresponds to a decrease in the visual span for vertical reading.

Chung demonstrated that perceptual learning can improve RSVP reading speed in people with AMD after training [82]. Face discrimination and recognition can also be reliably improved in patients with AMD using perceptual learning on face discrimination tasks [83]. Furthermore, Liu et al. [84], who trained people with severe visual impairment (due to different conditions, including AMD) on a visual search task, observed that both search speed and accuracy of the search improved after training, with the improvements being maintained for a period of time at least one month.

Pijnacker et al. [85] proposed to evaluate whether perceptual learning obtains similar results compared to eccentric vision training and oculomotor training, finding in all these interventions effective methods for reading rehabilitation in AMD patients. On the other hand, Seiple et al. [86] supported the efficacy of ocular movement control over eccentric viewing training and RSVP when compared to people with AMD, which does not imply considering the other methods as ineffective.

6. Modern technologies in VR

Digital technologies have improved reading opportunities for AMD patients, first by transferring the text to video screens where it can be manipulated and, more recently, in digital representations that can be personalized [87].

In this sense, several devices that such as CCTVs, tablets, smartphones, or electronic readers have shown a great potential to improve reading ability in individuals with CFL.

One of these technologies whose effectiveness in improving reading between CFL patients has been clinically proven is the iPad (**Figure 6**). This was demonstrated by a study in which, with the help of the character magnification provided by the iPad, 64 out of 73 patients with AMD (88%) were able to read standard size text (N8) or smaller [88].

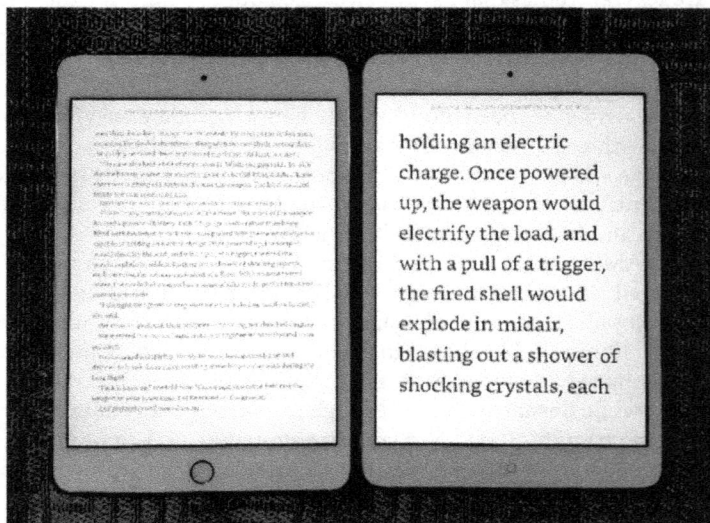

Figure 6.
Character magnification provided by the iPad [20].

Another study conducted in 100 patients with low vision (of whom 57 had AMD) found that the iPad offers read speed improvement performance comparable to CCTV systems and home magnification devices, making it a less costly and bulky option for visually impaired people seeking VR [89].

Within this line of work, several applications are being developed for implementation on such devices, such as the MD_evReader application, which scrolls text in a single line to improve reading performance by reducing the demands on the eye movement system and minimising the effects of perceptual crowding [90], proving to reduce reading error rates in individuals with CFL [91].

Modern technologies relevant to VR also include HMDs, which comprise a miniature electronic display in close proximity to one or both eyes which causes a highly magnified virtual image of the miniature screen to appear at a comfortable distance for the viewer. At the present moment, these devices have only demonstrated significant improvements in distance and intermediate visual acuity when compared to conventional optical LVAs in patients with AMD [92], but with the rapid evolution of virtual and augmented reality technologies, innovative approaches are making their way in this field.

For example, in a study which tested the effectiveness of a virtual bioptic telescope and a virtual projection screen implemented with an HMD, improvements in functional ability outcomes estimated from visual information, targets difficulty ratings and reading were observed in a sample of 30 patients with AMD and bilateral central scotomas [93].

Other noteworthy technologies in this area include portable artificial vision devices, such as The OrCam MyEye, which employs a miniature television camera mounted on the frame of the spectacles to recognize text, monetary denominations, faces, and other objects if activated by the patient pressing a trigger button, allowing people with visual impairment to understand text and identify objects through audio feedback. The device, which has recently been commercialized, has proven to be an effective tool for different low-vision patients, leading to contrasted improvements in several visual activities even superior to those achieved with previously used optical aids [94].

7. VR for mobility and ADLs

There is little scientific evidence of the impact of the use of eccentric viewing on ADLs and safe mobility. Some researchers have determined that development of PRL can occur naturally and that there may even be several PRLs used by the subject [95].

Vukicevic et al. conducted a study with 48 people diagnosed with AMD, aged 60 or over with visual acuity equal to or less than 20/200 (1.0 LogMAR unit) with the aim of investigating the impact of eccentric viewing training on daily self-care activities. To this end, two groups were formed, of which one received eccentric viewing training while the other did not [96]. The results show that even if the subjects had already established their PRL, the execution of daily life tasks improved.

In the case of ADLs, in addition to eccentric viewing training there are other factors that can significantly affect the performance of ADLs, such as lighting, familiarity with the environment, and contrast in materials and surroundings [97].

Illumination is an important method for improving the use of remanent vision, but there are differences between people as to what they consider adequate or comfortable. This is why specialists have to take into account not only the intensity and type of light, but also the surface on which it is to be applied and its position in relation to the subject, adapting it to the preferred viewing area [98].

In other words, being familiar with an environment, with the organization in space of its elements and the appropriate use of lighting can favor the use of PRL, and, hence, the execution of ADLs in an efficient manner.

Liu reviews interventional therapies to improve ADL performance and highlights that patients with AMD can benefit from vision training and the use of optical AVLs, but they need more than that; such as developing skills, using devices or learning problem-solving strategies, so intervention should be multidisciplinary and carried out in multiple sessions to give people enough time to adapt to new devices and skills [99].

Safe mobility for AMD patients is clearly conditioned by the risk of falls, which in the older population can lead to other serious consequences. Displacement in the elderly population is characterized by the involvement of different factors like balance, hearing, reaction capacity and decision-making. From the perspective of vision, the effects on the visual field, contrast sensitivity or the way in which lighting conditions affect the subject are determining factors in how the person will be able to travel [100]. It can be seen that, once again, there are multiple factors involved in the performance of this activity, which implies a multidisciplinary intervention and training in multiple sessions until adaptation to the new skills is achieved.

It is important to properly assess the visual field and information processing in this area in people with low vision, since the processing itself is more complex in detecting objects in the mobile environment while when using the microperimetry test only simple items are detected [101].

Eye and head searching movements when crossing are more difficult in AMD than in normally-sighted people, and there are no stable patterns as in reading. They also involve decision making such as the right time to cross, where the speed of walking among other aspects is crucial for safe movement and good decision making. To this must be add that, as mentioned, the ability to react in older people is diminished. Geruschat et al. confirms that patients with AMD present a higher risk due to increased latency when identifying the right moment to cross a street [102].

The optical devices that patients with AMD mainly use for mobility are telescopes; so are the filters as mentioned above. As for other activities, training and perceptual learning are presented as a decisive factor for the successful rehabilitation of patients with the aim of safe movement.

8. Conclusions

Although most researchers usually focus on studying eccentric viewing training in individuals with AMD, mainly for reading purposes, it cannot be forgotten that there are many aspects that explain visual functioning for any task. Therefore, research in VR has to consider the multifactorial intervention of characteristics such as the use of eccentric viewing training, the effect of crowding, the improvement of certain visual skills thanks to training during a certain period of time, as well as that of other factors that, although they are currently being studied in depth by authors such as Chung, still need more information to understand their real importance in VR.

Although there are few studies on the transfer of learning and training for reading to other ADLs and mobility, it can be said that visual training guarantees improvements in visual functioning for reading and other tasks, like face discrimination, recognition.

In addition to perceptual learning, oculomotor control and eccentric viewing training, other strategies that may improve reading ability in AMD patients include environmental changes (such as better lighting) and the prescription of filters and optical LVAs, such as high-plus reading lenses and different magnifiers (including clip-on, hand-held, or stand devices). Furthermore, many patients can also benefit from the use of electronic reading aids, including tablets, smartphones, electronic readers, HMDs or CCTV systems.

The widespread presence of accessible portable devices and software has led to a breakthrough in access to information and travel assistance for people with low vision. Some studies are therefore looking at the evidence for the use of such digital devices by the population, in contrast to the use of optical aids.

In fact, there is no such dilemma, because, as initially discussed, AMD patients are increasingly demanding a wider and more varied range of objectives to meet their needs, and the availability of a wider range of resources is only intended to meet these demands.

On the other hand, there are multiple factors involved in the visual skills that a person with AMD must perform, so a greater variety of resources offers the possibility of finding those best suited to their visual conditions.

Conflict of interest

The authors declare that there is no conflict of interest on the devices or technologies described in this chapter.

Abbreviations

ADLs	Activities of Daily Living
AMD	Age-Related Macular Degeneration
BCVA	Best-Corrected Visual Acuity
BFT	Biofeedback Fixation Training
CCTV	Closed-circuit Television
CFL	Central Field Loss
CNV	Choroidal Neovascularization
GA	Geographic Atrophy
HMDs	Head Mounted Displays
IMTs	Implantable Miniature Telescopes
LCD	Liquid-Crystal Display
LVAs	Low-Vision Aids
PRL	Preferred Retinal Locus
QoL	Quality of Life
RPE	Retinal Pigment Epithelium
RSVP	Rapid Serial Visual Presentation
VEGF	Vascular Endothelial Growth Factor
VR	Visual Rehabilitation
WHO	World Health Organization

Author details

Luis Leal Vega[1], Irene Alcoceba Herrero[1], Adrián Martín Gutiérrez[1*],
Joaquín Herrera Medina[2], Natalia Martín Cruz[3], Juan F. Arenillas Lara[4,5]
and María Begoña Coco Martín[1]

1 Group of Applied Clinical Neurosciences and Advanced Data Analysis,
Department of Medicine, Dermatology and Toxicology, Faculty of Medicine,
University of Valladolid, Valladolid, Spain

2 Group of Applied Clinical Neurosciences and Advanced Data Analysis,
Department of Surgery, Ophthalmology, Otolaryngology and Physiotherapy,
Faculty of Medicine, University of Valladolid, Valladolid, Spain

3 Group of Applied Clinical Neurosciences and Advanced Data Analysis,
Department of Business Organization and Marketing and Market Research,
Faculty of Economics and Business, University of Valladolid, Valladolid, Spain

4 Department of Medicine, University of Valladolid, Valladolid, Spain

5 Department of Neurology, Hospital Clínico Universitario, Valladolid, Spain

*Address all correspondence to: adrian.martn@gmail.com

IntechOpen

References

[1] Al-Zamil WM, Yassin SA. Recent developments in age-related macular degeneration: a review. Clinical Interventions in Aging. 2017;12:1313-1330. DOI: 10.2147/CIA.S143508

[2] Jonas JB. Global prevalence of age-related macular degeneration. Lancet Global Health. 2014;2(2):e65- 6. DOI: 10.1016/S2214-109X(13)70145-1

[3] Bourne RR, Stevens GA, et al; Vision Loss Expert Group. Causes of vision loss worldwide, 1990-2010: a systematic analysis. Lancet Global Health. 2013;1(6):e339-e349. DOI: 10.1016/S2214-109X(13)70113-X

[4] The International Council of Ophthalmology. The global economic cost of visual impairment [Internet]. Available from: http://www.icoph.org/resources/146/The-Global-Economic-Cost-of-Visual-Impairment.html [Accessed: 2020-12-01]

[5] Wong WL, et al. Global prevalence of age-related macular degeneration and disease burden projection for 2020 and 2040: a systematic review and meta-analysis. Lancet Glob Health. 2014;2(2):e106-e116. DOI: 10.1016/S2214-109X(13)70145-1

[6] Lim LS, Mitchell P, Seddon JM, Holz FG, Wong TY. Age-related macular degeneration. Lancet. 2012;379(9827):1728-1738. DOI: 10.1016/S0140-6736(12)60282-7

[7] Joachim N, Mitchell P, Burlutsky G, Kifley A, Wang JJ. The Incidence and Progression of Age-Related Macular Degeneration over 15 Years: The Blue Mountains Eye Study. Ophthalmology. 2015;122(12):2482-2489. DOI: 10.1016/j.ophtha.2015.08.002

[8] Mitchell P, Liew G, Gopinath B, Wong TY. Age-related macular degeneration. Lancet. 2018;392(10153):1147-1159. DOI: 10.1016/S0140-6736(18)31550-2

[9] Age-Related Eye Disease Study Research Group. Risk factors associated with age-related macular degeneration. A case-control study in the age-related eye disease study. Ophthalmology. 2000;107(12):2224-32. DOI: 10.1016/s0161-6420(00)00409-7

[10] Zarbin MA. Current concepts in the pathogenesis of age-related macular degeneration. 2004;122(4):598-614. DOI: 10.1001/archopht.122.4.598

[11] Zhang M, et al. Dysregulated metabolic pathways in age-related macular degeneration. Scientific Reports. 2020;10:2464. DOI: 10.1038/s41598-020-59244-4

[12] Datta S, et al. The impact of oxidative stress and inflammation on RPE degeneration in non-neovascular AMD. Progress in Retinal and Eye Research. 2017;60:201-218. DOI: 10.1016/j.preteyeres.2017.03.002

[13] EYE-RISK consortium; European Eye Epidemiology (E3) consortium. Prevalence of Age-Related Macular Degeneration in Europe: The Past and the Future. Ophthalmology. 2017;124(12):1753-1763. DOI: 10.1016/j.ophtha.2017.05.035

[14] Claessen H, et al. Evidence for a considerable decrease in total and cause-specific incidences of blindness in Germany. European Journal of Epidemiology. 2012;27(7):519-524 DOI: 10.1007/s10654-012-9705-7

[15] Age-Related Eye Disease Study 2 Research Group. Lutein + zeaxanthin and omega-3 fatty acids for age-related macular degeneration: Age-Related Eye Disease Study 2 (AREDS2) randomized clinical trial. JAMA. 2013;309(19):2005-15. DOI: 10.1001/jama.2013.4997

[16] Evans JR, Lawrenson JG. Antioxidant vitamin and mineral supplements for preventing age-related macular degeneration. The Cochrane Database of Systematic Reviews. 2017;7(7):CD000253. DOI: 10.1002/14651858.CD000253.pub4

[17] Andreoli CM, Miller JW. Anti-vascular endothelial growth factor therapy for ocular neovascular disease. Current Opinion in Ophthalmology. 2007;18(6):502-508. DOI: 10.1097/ICU.0b013e3282f0ca54

[18] Taylor DJ, Hobby AE, Binns AM, Crabb DP. How does age-related macular degeneration affect real-world visual ability and quality of life? A systematic review. BMJ Open. 2016;6(12):e011504. DOI: 10.1136/bmjopen-2016-011504

[19] World Health Organization. International classification of functioning, disability and health: ICF [Internet]. Available from: ea54r21.pdf (who.int) [Accessed: 2020-12-11]

[20] Colenbrander A. Vision Rehabilitation is Part of AMD Care. Vision (Basel). 2018;2(1):4. DOI: 10.3390/vision2010004

[21] Markowitz SN. Principles of modern low vision rehabilitation. Canadian Journal of Ophthalmology. 2006;41(3):289-312. DOI: 10.1139/I06-027

[22] Wilkinson ME, Shahid KS. Low vision rehabilitation: An update. Saudi Journal of Ophthalmology. 2018;32(2):134-138. DOI: 10.1016/j.sjopt.2017.10.005

[23] Lorenzini MC, Wittich W. Factors related to the use of magnifying low vision aids: a scoping review. Disability and Rehabilitation. 2020;42(24):3525-3537. DOI: 10.1080/09638288.2019.1593519

[24] Cheong AM, Lovie-Kitchin JE, Bowers AR, et al. Short-term in-office practice improves reading performance with stand magnifiers for people with AMD. Optometry and Vision Science. 2005;82(2):114-127. DOI: 10.1097/01.opx.0000153244.93582.ff

[25] Coco-Martín MB, Cuadrado-Asensio R, et al. Design and evaluation of a customized reading rehabilitation program for patients with age-related macular degeneration. Ophthalmology. 2013;120(1):151-159. DOI: 10.1016/j.ophtha.2012.07.035

[26] Kaltenegger K, Kuester S, et al. Effects of home reading training on reading and quality of life in AMD-a randomized and controlled study. Graefe's Archive for Clinical and Experimental Ophthalmology. 2019;257(7):1499-1512. DOI: 10.1007/s00417-019-04328-9

[27] Stelmack JA, Tang XC, Wei Y, Wilcox DT, Morand T, Brahm K, Sayers S, et al; LOVIT II Study Group. Outcomes of the Veterans Affairs Low Vision Intervention Trial II (LOVIT II): A Randomized Clinical Trial. JAMA Ophthalmology. 2017;135(2):96-104. DOI: 10.1001/jamaophthalmol.2016.4742

[28] Elliott DB, et al. Demographic characteristics of the vision-disabled elderly. Investigative Ophthalmology and Visual Sciences. 1997;38(12):2566-2575.

[29] Chung STL. Reading in the presence of macular disease: a mini-review. Ophthalmic and Physiological Optics. 2020;40(2):171-186. DOI: 10.1111/opo.12664

[30] Tarita-Nistor L, Brent MH, Steinbach MJ, et al. Fixation stability during binocular viewing in patients with age-related macular degeneration. Investigative Ophthalmology & Visual

Science. 2011;52(3):1887-1893. DOI: 10.1167/iovs.10-6059

[31] Schuchard RA. Preferred retinal loci and macular scotoma characteristics in patients with age-related macular degeneration. Canadian Journal of Ophthalmology. 2005;40(3):303-312. DOI: 10.1016/S0008-4182(05)80073-0

[32] Rubin GS. Measuring reading performance. Vision Research. 2013;90:43-51. DOI: 10.1016/j.visres.2013.02.015

[33] Denniss J, Baggaley HC, et al. Properties of Visual Field Defects Around the Monocular Preferred Retinal Locus in Age-Related Macular Degeneration. Investigative Ophthalmology & Visual Science. 2017;58(5):2652-2658. DOI: 10.1167/iovs.16-21086

[34] Markowitz M, Daibert-Nido M, Markowitz SN. Rehabilitation of reading skills in patients with age-related macular degeneration. Canadian Journal of Ophthalmology. 2018;53(1):3-8. DOI: 10.1016/j.jcjo.2017.10.042

[35] MacKeben M, et al. Effects Of Ranibizumab Injections On Functional Vision In Advanced Amd. Investigative Ophthalmology & Visual Science. 2012;53(14):4395.

[36] Fletcher DC, Mackeben M. Everyday use of modern microperimetry in a low-vision service. Canadian Journal of Ophthalmology. 2013;48(5):e99-e101. DOI: 10.1016/j.jcjo.2013.03.025

[37] Crossland MD, et al. Preferred retinal locus development in patients with macular disease. Ophthalmology. 2005;112(9):1579-1585. DOI: 10.1016/j.ophtha.2005.03.027

[38] Hassan SE, Ross NC, et al. Changes in the Properties of the Preferred

Retinal Locus with Eccentric Viewing Training. Optometry and Vision Science. 2019;96(2):79-86. DOI: 10.1097/OPX.0000000000001324

[39] Rubin GS. Vision rehabilitation for patients with age-related macular degeneration. Eye. 2001;15(Pt 3):430-435. DOI: 10.1038/eye.2001.148

[40] Nilsson UL, Frennesson C, Nilsson SE. Patients with AMD and a large absolute central scotoma can be trained successfully to use eccentric viewing, as demonstrated in a scanning laser ophthalmoscope. Vision Research. 2003;43(16):1777-1787. DOI: 10.1016/s0042-6989(03)00219-0

[41] Palmer S, Logan D, et al. Effective rehabilitation of reading by training in the technique of eccentric viewing: evaluation of a 4-year programme of service delivery. British Journal of Ophthalmology. 2010;94(4):494-497. DOI: 10.1136/bjo.2008.152231

[42] Hamade N, Hodge WG, Rakibuz-Zaman M, et al. The Effects of Low-Vision Rehabilitation on Reading Speed and Depression in Age Related Macular Degeneration: A Meta-Analysis. PLoS One. 2016;11(7):e0159254. DOI: 10.1371/journal.pone.0159254

[43] Watson GR, et al. Effects of preferred retinal locus placement on text navigation and development of advantageous trained retinal locus. Journal of Rehabilitation Research & Development. 2006;43(6):761-770. DOI: 10.1682/jrrd.2005.07.0120

[44] Cheong AM, Legge GE, et al. Relationship between slow visual processing and reading speed in people with macular degeneration. Vision research, 47(23), 2943-2955. DOI: 10.1016/j.visres.2007.07.010

[45] Chung ST, Legge GE, et al. Letter-recognition and reading speed

in peripheral vision benefit from perceptual learning. Vision Research. 2004;44(7):695-709. DOI: 10.1016/j.visres.2003.09.028

[46] Crossland MD, Culham LE, Rubin GS. Predicting reading fluency in patients with macular disease. Optometry and Vision Science. 2005;82(1):11-17.

[47] Xiong YZ, et al. Relationship Between Acuity and Contrast Sensitivity: Differences Due to Eye Disease. Investigative Ophthalmology & Visual Science. 2020;61(6):40. DOI: 10.1167/iovs.61.6.40

[48] Arditi A. Improving the design of the letter contrast sensitivity test. Investigative Ophthalmology & Visual Science. 2005;46(6):2225-2229. DOI: 10.1167/iovs.04-1198

[49] Haymes SA, Lee J. Effects of task lighting on visual function in age-related macular degeneration. Ophthalmic and Physiological Optics. 2006;26(2):169-179. DOI: 10.1111/j.1475-1313.2006.00367.x

[50] Bowers AR, Meek C, Stewart N. Illumination and reading performance in age-related macular degeneration. Clinical & Experimental Optometry. 2001;84(3):139-147. DOI: 10.1111/j.1444-0938.2001.tb04957.x

[51] Seiple W, Overbury O, et al. Effects of Lighting on Reading Speed as a Function of Letter Size. American Journal of Occupational Therapy. 2018;72(2):7202345020p1-72023450 20p7. DOI: 10.5014/ajot.2018.021873

[52] Chung ST. The effect of letter spacing on reading speed in central and peripheral vision. Investigative Ophthalmology and Visual Science. 2002;43(4):1270-1276. DOI: 10.1097/00006324-200012001-00034

[53] Chung ST, Jarvis SH, Woo SY, Hanson K, Jose RT. Reading speed does not benefit from increased line spacing in AMD patients. Optometry and Vision Science. 2008;85(9):827-833. DOI: 10.1097/OPX.0b013e31818527ea

[54] Wolffsohn JS, Dinardo C, Vingrys AJ. Benefit of coloured lenses for age-related macular degeneration. Ophthalmic and Physiological Optics. 2002;22(4):300-311. DOI: 10.1046/j.1475-1313.2002.00036.x

[55] Boucart M, Despretz P, Hladiuk K, Desmettre T. Does context or color improve object recognition in patients with low vision? Visual Neuroscience. 2008;25(5-6):685-689. DOI: 10.1017/S0952523808080826

[56] Brunnström G, Sörensen S, et al. Quality of light and quality of life-the effect of lighting adaptation among people with low vision. Ophthalmic and Physiological Optics. 2004;24(4):274-280. DOI: 10.1111/j.1475-1313.2004.00192.x

[57] Caballe-Fontanet D, Alvarez-Peregrina C, et al. Improvement of the Quality of Life in Patients with Age-Related Macular Degeneration by Using Filters. International Journal of Environmental Research and Public Health. 2020;17(18),6751. DOI: 10.3390/ijerph17186751

[58] Christoforidis JB, Tecce N, Dell'Omo R, Mastropasqua R, et al. Age-related macular degeneration and visual disability. Current Drug Targets. 2011;12(2):221-233. DOI: 10.2174/138945011794182755

[59] Virgili G, Acosta R, Bentley SA, Giacomelli G, et al. Reading aids for adults with low vision. The Cochrane Database Systematic Review. 2018;4(4):CD003303. DOI: 10.1002/14651858.CD003303.pub4

[60] Shah P, Schwartz SG, et al. Low vision services: a practical guide for the clinician. Therapeutic

Advances in Ophthalmology. 2018;10:2515841418776264. DOI: 10.1177/2515841418776264

[61] Khan SA, Das T, Kumar SM, Nutheti R. Low vision rehabilitation in patients with age-related macular degeneration at a tertiary eye care centre in southern India. Clinical & Experimental Ophthalmology. 2002;30(6):404-410. DOI: 10.1046/j.1442-9071.2002.00569.x

[62] Brinker BP, Beek PJ. Reading with magnifiers. Ergonomics. 1996;39(10):1231-1248. DOI: 10.1080/00140139608964542

[63] Spitzberg LA, Goodrich GL. New ergonomic stand magnifiers. Journal of the American Optometry Association. 1995;66(1):25-30.

[64] Maghami MH, Sodagar AM, et al. Visual prostheses: the enabling technology to give sight to the blind. Journal of Ophthalmic and Vision Research. 2014;9(4):494-505. DOI: 10.4103/2008-322X.150830

[65] Lane SS, Kuppermann BD, Fine IH, et al. A prospective multicenter clinical trial to evaluate the safety and effectiveness of the implantable miniature telescope. American Journal of Ophthalmology. 2004;137(6):993-1001. DOI: 10.1016/j.ajo.2004.01.030

[66] IMT-002 Study Group. Implantable miniature telescope for the treatment of visual acuity loss resulting from end-stage age-related macular degeneration: 1-year results. Ophthalmology. 2006;113(11):1987-2001. DOI: 10.1016/j.ophtha.2006.07.010

[67] IMT002 Study Group. Implantable telescope for end-stage age-related macular degeneration: long-term visual acuity and safety outcomes. American Journal of Ophthalmology. 2008;146(5):664-673. DOI: 10.1016/j.ajo.2008.07.003

[68] Nguyen N, Weismann M, et al. Improvement of reading speed after providing of low vision aids in patients with age-related macular degeneration. Acta Ophthalmologica. 2009;87(8):849-853. DOI: 10.1111/j.1755-3768.2008.01423.x

[69] Jackson ML, Schoessow KA, Selivanova A, et al. Adding access to a video magnifier to standard vision rehabilitation: initial results on reading performance and well-being from a prospective, randomized study. Digital Journal of Ophthalmology. 201731;23(1):1-10. DOI: 10.5693/djo.01.2017.02.001

[70] Taylor JJ, Bambrick R, Brand A, et al. Effectiveness of portable electronic and optical magnifiers for near vision activities in low vision: a randomized crossover trial. Ophthalmic and Physiological Optics. 2017;37(4):370-384. DOI: 10.1111/opo.12379

[71] Ehrlich JR, et al. Head-Mounted Display Technology for Low-Vision Rehabilitation and Vision Enhancement. American Journal of Ophthalmology. 2017;176:26-32. DOI: 10.1016/j.ajo.2016.12.021

[72] Crossland MD, Macedo AF, Rubin GS. Electronic books as low vision aids. British Journal of Ophthalmology. 2010;94(8):1109. DOI: 10.1136/bjo.2009.170167

[73] Crossland MD, Silva RS, et al. Smartphone, tablet computer and e-reader use by people with vision impairment. Ophthalmic and Physiological Optics. 2014;34(5):552-557. DOI: 10.1111/opo.12136

[74] Barraza-Bernal MJ, et al. A preferred retinal location of fixation can be induced when systematic stimulus relocations are applied. Journal of Vision. 2017;17(2):11. DOI: 10.1167/17.2.11

[75] Morales MU, et al. Biofeedback fixation training method for improving eccentric vision in patients with loss of foveal function secondary to different maculopathies. International Ophthalmology. 2020;40:305-312. DOI: 10.1007/s10792-019-01180-y

[76] Liu R, Kwon M. Integrating oculomotor and perceptual training to induce a pseudo fovea: A model system for studying central vision loss. Journal of Vision. 2016;16(6):10. DOI: 10.1167/16.6.10

[77] Legge GE, et al. Psychophysics of reading: XX. Linking letter recognition to reading speed in central and peripheral vision. Vision Research. 2001;41(6):725-743. DOI: 10.1016/S0042-6989(00)00295-9

[78] Zhu Z, Hu Y, Liao C, Huang R, et al. Perceptual Learning of Visual Span Improves Chinese Reading Speed. Investigative Ophthalmology & Visual Science. 2019;60(6):2357-2368. DOI: 10.1167/iovs.18-25780

[79] Yu D, Cheung SH, et al. Reading speed in the peripheral visual field of older adults: Does it benefit from perceptual learning? Vision Research. 2010;50(9):860-869. DOI: 10.1016/j.visres.2010.02.006

[80] Bernard JB, Arunkumar A, Chung ST. Can reading-specific training stimuli improve the effect of perceptual learning on peripheral reading speed? Vision Research. 2012;66:17-25. DOI: 10.1016/j.visres.2012.06.012

[81] Yu D, Legge GE, Park H, Gage E, Chung ST. Development of a training protocol to improve reading performance in peripheral vision. Vision Research. 2011;50(1):36-45. DOI: 10.1016/j.visres.2009.10.005

[82] Chung ST. Improving Reading Speed for People with Central Vision Loss Through Perceptual Learning. Investigative Ophthalmology & Visual Science. 2011;52(2):1164-1170. DOI: 10.1167/iovs.10-6034

[83] Haris EM, McGraw PV, Webb BS, Chung STL, Astle AT. The Effect of Perceptual Learning on Face Recognition in Individuals with Central Vision Loss. Investigative Ophthalmology & Visual Science. 2011;52(2):1164-1170. DOI: 10.1167/iovs.61.8.2

[84] Liu L, Kuyk T, Fuhr P. Visual search training in subjects with severe to profound low vision. Vision Research. 2007;47(20):2627-2636. DOI: 10.1016/j.visres.2007.07.001

[85] Pijnacker J, et al. Rehabilitation of reading in older individuals with macular degeneration: a review of effective training programs. Neuropsychology, Development and Cognition, Section B, Aging, Neuropsychology and Cognition. 2011;18(6):708-732. DOI: 10.1080/13825585.2011.613451

[86] Seiple W, Grant P, Szlyk JP. Reading rehabilitation of individuals with AMD: relative effectiveness of training approaches. Investigative Ophthalmology & Visual Science. 2011;52(6):2938-2944. DOI: 10.1167/iovs.10-6137

[87] Granquist C, Wu YH, Gage R, Crossland MD, et al. How People with Low Vision Achieve Magnification in Digital Reading. Optometry and Vision Science. 2018;95(9):711-719. DOI: 10.1097/OPX.0000000000001261

[88] Haji SA, Sambhav K, Grover S, Chalam KV. Evaluation of the iPad as a low vision aid for improving reading ability. Clinical Ophthalmology. 2014;9:17-20. DOI: 10.2147/OPTH.S73193

[89] Morrice E, Johnson AP, Marinier JA, Wittich W. Assessment of the Apple

iPad as a low-vision reading aid. Eye. 2017;31(6):865-871. DOI: 10.1038/eye.2016.309

[90] Walker R. An iPad app as a low-vision aid for people with macular disease. British Journal of Ophthalmology. 2013;97(1):110-112. DOI: 10.1136/bjophthalmol-2012-302415

[91] Walker R, Bryan L, et al. The value of Tablets as reading aids for individuals with central visual field loss: an evaluation of eccentric reading with static and scrolling text. Ophthalmic and Physiological Optics. 2016;36(4):459-464. DOI: 10.1111/opo.12296

[92] Culham LE, et al. Clinical performance of electronic, head-mounted, low-vision devices. Ophthalmic and Physiological Optics. 2004;24(4):281-290. DOI: 10.1111/j.1475-1313.2004.00193.x

[93] Deemer AD, Swenor BK, Fujiwara K, Deremeik JT, Ross NC, et al. Preliminary Evaluation of Two Digital Image Processing Strategies for Head-Mounted Magnification for Low Vision Patients. Translational Vision Science & Technology. 2019;8(1):23. DOI: 10.1167/tvst.8.1.23

[94] Moisseiev E, Mannis MJ. Evaluation of a Portable Artificial Vision Device Among Patients With Low Vision. JAMA Ophthalmology. 2016;134(7):748-752. DOI: 10.1001/jamaophthalmol.2016.1000

[95] Fletcher DC, Schuchard RA. Preferred retinal loci relationship to macular scotomas in a low-vision population. Ophthalmology. 1997;104(4):632-638. DOI: 10.1016/s0161-6420(97)30260-7

[96] Vukicevic M, et al. Eccentric Viewing Training in the Home Environment: Can it Improve the

Performance of Activities of Daily Living? Journal of Visual Impairment & Blindness. 2009;103(5):277-290. DOI: 10.1177/0145482X0910300506

[97] Colenbrander A, Fletcher DC. Contrast Sensitivity and ADL Performance. Investigative Ophthalmology & Visual Science. 2006;47(13): 5834.

[98] Corn AL, Erin JN. Foundations of low vision: Clinical and functional perspectives. New York: AFB Press. 2010.

[99] Liu CJ, Brost MA, et al. Occupational therapy interventions to improve performance of daily activities at home for older adults with low vision: a systematic review. The American Journal of Occupational Therapy. 2013;67(3):279-287. DOI: 10.5014/ajot.2013.005512

[100] Trauzettel-Klosinski S. Current methods of visual rehabilitation. Deutsches Ärzteblatt International. 2011;108(51-52),871-878. DOI: 10.3238/arztebl.2011.0871

[101] Tadin D, Nyquist JB, et al. Peripheral vision of youths with low vision: motion perception, crowding, and visual search. Investigative Ophthalmology & Visual science. 2012;53(9):5860-5868. DOI: 10.1167/iovs.12-10350

[102] Geruschat DR, Fujiwara K, Emerson RS. Traffic gap detection for pedestrians with low vision. Optometry and Vision Science. 2011;88(2):208-216. DOI: 10.1097/OPX.0b013e3182045988

www.ingramcontent.com/pod-product-compliance
Lightning Source LLC
Chambersburg PA
CBHW081224190326
41458CB00016B/5674